Advances in Experimental Medicine and Biology

Clinical and Experimental Biomedicine

Volume 1335

More information about this series at http://www.springer.com/subseries/16003

Mieczyslaw Pokorski
Editor

Best Practice in Health Care

Springer

Editor
Mieczyslaw Pokorski
The Jan Dlugosz University
Częstochowa, Poland

ISSN 0065-2598 ISSN 2214-8019 (electronic)
Advances in Experimental Medicine and Biology
ISSN 2523-3769 ISSN 2523-3777 (electronic)
Clinical and Experimental Biomedicine
ISBN 978-3-030-77741-8 ISBN 978-3-030-77742-5 (eBook)
https://doi.org/10.1007/978-3-030-77742-5

This Springer imprint is published by the registered company Springer Nature Switzerland AG
The registered company address is: Gewerbestrasse 11, 6330 Cham, Switzerland

Contents

Adv Exp Med Biol - Clinical and Experimental Biomedicine (2022) 13: 1–10
https://doi.org/10.1007/5584_2021_620

Published online: 26 March 2021

Artificial Intelligence in the Healthcare System: An Overview

Jacek Lorkowski, Oliwia Grzegorowska, and Mieczysław Pokorski

Abstract

This chapter aims to present insights into the influence of artificial intelligence (AI) on medicine, public health, and the economy. PubMed and Google Scholar databases were used for the identification and collection of articles with search commands of "artificial intelligence" AND "public health" and "artificial intelligence" AND "medicine". A total of 273 articles specifically handling the issue of artificial intelligence, dating ten years back, in three major medical journals: *Science*, *The Lancet*, and *The New England Journal of Medicine*, were analyzed. Computational power gets stronger by the day, giving us new solutions and possibilities. Current medicine problems like personalized medicine, storage of data, and documentation overload will likely be replaced by AI shortly. The application of AI may also bring substantial benefits to other areas of medicine like the diagnostic and therapeutic processes. The development and spread of AI are inescapable as it lowers healthcare and administrative costs, improves medical efficiency, and predicts and prevents major disease complications. The use of AI in medicine seems destined to carry the day.

Keywords

Artificial intelligence · Healthcare system · Medical documentation · Medicine · Public health

1 Introduction

Astronomy is probably the first field in which openness in sharing the knowledge brought about the milestone progress for man as the notes of Chinese astronomers dated to 1054 AD enabled Carlo Otto Lampland to discover a remnant of the supernova Crab Nebula in 1921 (Fore 2019). The faith in the progress achieved through cooperation and parallel learning helps achieve success, even if it is a collaboration between distant generations. Likewise, in high-energy physics, access to open data is essential for further discoveries and scientific progress. Large international scientific organizations, for instance, the

J. Lorkowski (✉)
Department of Orthopedics, Traumatology and Sports Medicine, Central Clinical Hospital of the Ministry of Internal Affairs and Administration, Warsaw, Poland

Faculty of Health Sciences, Medical University of Mazovia, Warsaw, Poland

O. Grzegorowska
Department of Cardiology, Independent Public Regional Hospital, Szczecin, Poland

M. Pokorski
Faculty of Health Sciences, The Jan Długosz University in Częstochowa, Częstochowa, Poland

Institute of Health Sciences, Opole University, Opole, Poland
e-mail: m.pokorski@ujd.edu.pl

European Council for Nuclear Research (CERN), founded in Europe in 1952, have become world-class research bodies by sharing knowledge with the global community. This is a progressive way of science practice based on cooperation rather than pure competition posed to bring about great discoveries.

A steady increase in the amount of data to be converted into knowledge enforces adequate software solutions, workflow, and explanations (Chen et al. 2019). To process petabytes of data, it is of the highest need to implement solutions of artificial intelligence (AI) because the work cannot be performed by a man (Lorkowski and Malinowska 2020). The introduction of such solutions is unavoidable, especially during the SARS-CoV-2 pandemic, when the time seems increasingly essential. The pandemic has hastened up this process. The AI and deep neural networks (DNN), designed for the analysis and processing of tremendous volumes of data, appear of critical help in drug or vaccine discoveries, observation of clinical effects, and further outcomes (Grzegorowska and Lorkowski 2020).

The 1970s can be considered as the onset of AI and knowledge sharing ideas in the modern world. The oil crisis of the time forced Jack Niles to propose the terms "teleworking" and "telecommuting" to reduce fuel consumption in the United States. Based on this innovative concept, Alvin Toeffler raised the idea of an electronic village as the main place of production in the future. The idea was broadly discussed in Europe, especially in Scandinavian countries, but the concept of telework was nearly forgotten. Then, it came back to life in the 1980s and is steadily on the rise since (Dangelmeier et al. 1999). The current SARS-CoV-2 pandemic situation has made this concept come true as people have started working from home due mostly to social distancing.

Biomedical science focuses on four interrelated topics: personalized medicine, data-intensive technologies, big data and information technologies, and AI (Schork 2019). This chapter aims to present a short insight into connections between artificial intelligence, medicine, public health, and the economy. To this end, we screened PubMed and Google Scholar databases using the commands of "artificial intelligence" AND "public health" and "artificial intelligence" AND "medicine". As of December 1, 2020, the search returned 18,000 and 11,000 entries concerning either combination terms, respectively, dating ten years back. From this huge volume of articles, we chose for further analyses those which specifically handled the issue of AI and were published in the following three renowned medical journals: 185 articles in *Science*, 61 in *The Lancet*, and 27 in *The New England Journal of Medicine*.

2 Public Health and Smart Cities

Charles Edward Amory Winslow of Yale University in New Haven, Connecticut, proposed the following definition of public health in 1920: "Public Health is the science and the art of preventing disease, prolonging life, and promoting physical health and efficiency through organized community efforts for the sanitation of the environment, the control of community infections, the education of the individual in principles of personal hygiene, the organization of medical and nursing service for the early diagnosis and preventive treatment of disease, and the development of the social machinery which will ensure to every individual in the community a standard of living adequate for the maintenance of health; organizing these benefits in such fashion as to enable every citizen to realize his birth right of health and longevity" (Winslow 1920). Public health uses specific methods and concepts to measure and describe health conditions. A widely used concept is the quality of life (QoL) is defined by the WHO as "individuals' perception of their position in the life in the context of the culture in which they live and in relation to their goals, expectations, standards, and concerns". The QoL is commonly evaluated in patients with cancer, mental illness, heart disease, gastrointestinal disease, chronic obstructive pulmonary disease, asthma, and in the elderly (Haraldstad et al. 2019). Public health sciences also explore how urbanization affects human life and health and to what extent citizens can influence their living conditions. It is known that city-dwelling relates to a better QoL, physical health, access to the healthcare system, as well as enabling the elderly to have better social and physical activities (Zagozdzon et al. 2011; Eggebeen and Lichter 1993). Such factors appear to entice people to dwell in big cities or their neighborhoods, which spurred the development of the 2003 New Charter of Athens, an innovative project connected to urbanization (Stouten 2003). From the healthcare standpoint, the purpose of such initiative has been to form a national health-promoting living space for residents by the reorganization of urban planning, inclusive of an entire range of public health services based on the use of information and communication technologies (ICT) (Lorkowski and Malinowska 2020). The ICT is involved in the prevention of life-threatening situations like cardiorespiratory arrest, cardiac and brain infarcts, accidental falls suffered by the frail elderly, and others requiring sophisticated and prompt help. These situations shape the idea of a smart city proposed by the International Communication Union and defined as "an innovative city that uses the ICT and other means to improve QoL, the efficiency of urban operations, and services, and competitiveness while ensuring that it meets the needs of present and future generations with respect to economic, social, and environmental aspects" (Toh et al. 2020). It follows that the use of AI is naturally integrated into the concept of a smart city. The United Kingdom, China, and India are the countries that have allocated substantial fiscal resources to design and implement smart cities (Toh et al. 2020).

The 2017 Global Smart City Performance Index, evaluating the four most important vectors in the city function such as mobility, healthcare, safety, and productivity, was topped by Singapore followed by London and New York (Smart Cities Association 2017). These cities ranked best on the number of hospital beds per capita, road security, air pollution, bicycle communication, public transport, telemedicine, digital health portals, virtual medical advisor assistance, elderly care, and campaigns promoting healthy ways of life. There are reports that each citizen "gets back" 15 days' worth of time every year owing to the ICT. This time can be spent on physical activity or sleep or adoption of healthy eating habits, which all positively affect cardio-cerebrovascular health (Riggs et al. 2018; Seixas et al. 2018). Physical activity reduces weight and glucose level and improves the quality of sleep, making also chronic obstructive pulmonary disease (COPD) patients benefit from it (Lewthwaite et al. 2017). The Global Liveability Index (2021) created by *The Economist* ranks 140 major cities in the categories of stability, culture and environment, education, infrastructure, and healthcare. Healthcare is evaluated in the smart city context by assessing both public and private systems. In 2018, the maximum score in the index was achieved by the cities of Vienna, Melbourne, Osaka, Calgary, Sydney, Vancouver, Toronto, Tokyo, and Adelaide.

On the other hand, the contemporary SARS-CoV-2 pandemic points out some limitations inherent to the smart city concept. One of them is the problem of communication systems as they are fragmented and often understood only by service providers. An effort should be made to standardize and find the best solution to cooperate in the case of disasters and comprehensively build cities regarding public health, particularly when the situation enforces social distancing or other extraordinary measures (Allam and Jones 2020; Capolongo et al. 2020).

3 Artificial Intelligence (AI)

AI is used in various fields, from public health to biology, and can be reduced to the task of predicting an outcome from diverse features or finding repeating patterns in large datasets (Deo 2015). Today, AI is mostly applicable in machine learning (ML), also in medicine. There are three kinds of ML—supervised, unsupervised, and reinforcement learning. When the first one focuses on the classification of the data, the second is trying to find unique patterns and assess their viability. The patterns are then evaluated in supervised learning tasks. Reinforcement learning is reward-based learning used mostly in robotic applications (Aktolun 2019). The most widely used method is supervised learning that uses the following algorithms: linear and logistic regressions, artificial neuron networks (ANN), support vector machines (SVM), and tree-based methods; all can be combined. A special subset of ML is the deep learning that builds the ANN, the process inspired by neural interconnections in the human brain and consisting of multiple layers made of nodes. The nodes are interconnected with nodes in the back and forward layers as it takes place in the brain. In practice, these methods help analyze huge amounts of data in a chosen context. The SVM builds a model that assigns new items to a category in the linear classification. Applying a kernel trick allows making nonlinear classifications by mapping their inputs into high-dimensional feature spaces. Finally, a decision tree is the most common method that reconstructs the tree structure and assigns labels by creating appropriate "splits" (Al'Aref et al. 2019).

AI is a strong technological sequence providing sources of machine deduction, reasoning, learning, and interaction. It has entered our everyday life by solving business problems sensibly and acceptably, including building advanced algorithms, analyzing data, enhancing the computational power and storage, and lowering costs (Ergen 2019). Despite these facts, AI has been portrayed by Stephen Hawking as a possible threat to the world economy as it may one day replace humanity. Also, people should focus on creating a beneficial AI rather than any AI, which is of essential importance for AI not to become a digitalized utopia (Hawking 2015).

4 Blockchain Technologies

The WHO has proposed a classification of digital healthcare services into interventions for clients, healthcare providers, health system or resource managers, and data services. We are currently a part of digital transformation where digital medical networks can be created using two different concepts. The first concept assumes the use of a centralized network, a technology tested during the First Gulf War and then used by corporations such as IBM and Walmart, which substantially increased profits and helped improve the quality of customer services. Referring to the medical field, a basic issue is to develop a centralized network that would be a fast and effective information exchange platform that ensures the security of data (Lorkowski and Malinowska 2020). The second concept, which gains popularity and progresses promptly, relates to the development of cryptocurrencies. It is the blockchain technology that enables transactions between two or more parties without a centralized authority and secures them with cryptographic principles making them inexpensive and fast. This technology can be defined as a chain of blocks with time stamps connected through cryptographic hashes. The chain can grow all the time as new blocks are added, with each new block containing a link to the content of a preceding block's link. The blockchain, called the distributed general ledger, is the distributed database, also known as the registry or common register. Each piece of information is stored as an independent copy of the registry on computers and servers around the world. It means that every user has its copy of all collected data (Kuo et al. 2017).

Key benefits of the blockchain, when compared to traditional databases for biomedical and healthcare applications, include decentralization and cryptography providing security and privacy in addition to immutability (data once saved cannot be changed, corrupted, or retrieved), assignment of health data to the patient, and data robustness, transparency, trust, and verifiability. This technology is used in electronic health records (EHR), remote patient monitoring, and pharmaceutical industries, where distributed data ledgers may improve the management of medical records and accelerate biomedical research and education. These fields also are vulnerable to potential threats of forgery.

Currently, a more patient-centered connection of different, previously independent noncommunication systems is needed, followed by transformation into reliable electronic databases. The development of blockchain networks in medicine is determined by connections between particular parts of the system. A major drawback is that these networks are created by different suppliers and based on different solutions, which creates compatibility and standardization problems. Another challenge is to adequately protect medical data against potential security breaches. Moreover, the European Union General Data Protection Regulation assumes that the user always has a right to request complete erasure of their data. The blockchain technology, on the other hand, makes it impossible due to immutability. Finally, very large volumes of data may degrade the processing performance by lowering the system's speed (Agbo et al. 2019).

5 Sensitive Data

A basic issue concerning a large collection of data and AI in medicine and public health is database safety. As data in medicine contain racial, genetic, biometric, and even religious belief information and evidence of identity, they are regarded as sensitive. That does not exclude the anonymous use of data, like in meta-analysis, which is a very worthwhile cause. Fortunately, the unauthorized use of sensitive data is unlikely when proper security measures are adopted. It happens some online applications have racial and socioeconomic denigrating content, which meets with public outcry. Such is usually introduced onto platforms through the commonly anonymized unfiltered data streaming from the Internet. Luckily, there have been no similar incidents in the healthcare system. However, further watchfulness and testing the security measures are required before full implementation of AI in healthcare (Al'Aref et al. 2019). Researchers argue that anonymization of medical data, particularly identity, is so well advanced that the security breach is less likely than gaining obtaining information from within the system due to the vulnerability of hospital records to external hacking. It means that the weakest link in the system may be a man. (Lorkowski and Malinowska 2020; Mearian 2018). The first AI-based and US Federal Drug Administration (FDA)-approved application for facilitating clinical, particularly cardiovascular, diagnoses, called the Arterys medical imaging platform, provides a unique solution for the Protected Health Information (PHI) service. The application splits out data that may be responsible for the evidence of identity and then stores them in the Arterys cloud and the hospital PHI secure server. These data can be later rebuilt when an accredited user logs into the system (Marr 2017).

Medical data are a potential economic resource for individuals, companies, and countries. The issue of sharing medical data remains unresolved as they should be processed in compliance with the highest ethical standards. Plausibly, a worldwide collection of medical data might be the most valuable and largest bunch of data humanity possesses. It might also become a potential global resource of strategic importance for humanity's development and prosperity. It all demands a special infrastructure, legal conditions, and making ways of collecting, processing, and storing of data, remembering to deal with the population data, not concerning individuals.

6 Medical Documentation

The volume of medical documentation increases every year, taking doctors' time away from the direct care of patients. This takes a toll on both physicians and patients and also increases the costs of medical services (Raulinajtys-Grzybek and Lorkowski 2020). A burnout syndrome, on the increase in physicians, appears connected with the time spent on filling and creating medical documentation. It has been estimated that each hour spent with a patient elates to two hours spent on EHR, mostly on documentation. In the United States, a "wasted" has been priced at 90–140 billion dollars in lost physician productivity every year (Lin 2020). It is known that there are two possibilities for creating and storing medical documentation: traditional on paper and digital. It is most probable that a mix of the two will persist for a long time to come. An unfortunate underestimation of the advantages of digitalized documentation is felt, which is an attempt to deny the laws of high numbers and statistics (Bloom and Cadarette 2019).

It is estimated that about 91 billion dollars (14% of public health spending) were wasted due to invalid administration in 2018. That pointedly shows that the current model of appointing principals and tasks for health bureaucracies simply does not work. Applying AI to provide an appropriate execution of operations and optimization of procedures should contribute to reductions in costs and lost opportunities. The excessive paperwork is a consequence of unreasonable and often reprised document circulation. Jonathan Bush has described this phenomenon as "sewage" of modern medicine, and applying AI for the analysis of bureaucratic procedures will reduce, improve, and redirect to the useful operational tracks. A reorganization of funds allocation, reduction of costs of lost opportunities, and the optimal cash flow are the most expected results of these actions. For many observers, the hitherto system of medical documentation in healthcare is seen as a huge, monolithic, difficult to use, and reform-inert structure. Paradoxically, the world's most popular systems of archiving data are often built based on old technologies that have been primarily dedicated to building first databases. That might be a reason they seem more intuitive for an average user (Bush and Baker 2014).

In an article published by *The New Yorker*, the implementation and evaluation of new software are time-consuming. Additionally, it needs constant improvements. A software system described was created not for the medical staff but for patients who would like to check their laboratory results, remember the drug list, or track their conditions. Any step forward toward more convenient patient-oriented management is beneficial from the medical and economic standpoints as the chances of health improvement and prompt return to work increase (Gawande 2018).

Creating the EHR helps streamline the patient visit. However, EHR affects the patient-physician communication in complex ways, enforcing changes in the consultation attitude that would satisfy both sides (Crampton et al. 2016). Medical Scribe services gain popularity, offering a smooth transition from speech into a written text, performing documentation in the EHR, and partnering with the physician to deliver the most efficient patient care (Ash et al. 2020). There also exist government-sponsored EHRs introduced to collect medical data from a wide range of people. Their main purpose is to monitor long-term clinical and public health patterns that might be therapeutically and epidemiologically useful for the future. The Biobank in the United Kingdom and the NIH *All of Us* Research Program in the United States of America change the practice of personalized medicine by collecting and evaluating data from millions of people to accelerate research, diagnosis, and treatment services (Bycroft et al. 2018; Sankar and Parker 2017).

Medical data are specific and heterogeneous and come in a variety of forms that are essential for proper identification of patient health status. Machine learning, which is capable of extracting information from data, is of substantial help in medical care. Large amounts of collected data require special processing to be introduced into AI algorithms that must be able to validate the information before its clinical adoption. That is why learning from and making predictions on data requires to split them into training, validation, and test sets. Test data should be prepared in a specific objective way, contain data from various hospitals and institutions, and used as often as possible (Park et al. 2019).

7 Multiomics, Precision, and Personalized Medicine

The biological identity is made of features characterized by individual epigenomics, genomics, metabolomics, microbiomics, pharmacogenomics, proteomics, and other "omic data", which all create a "permutome". The field has been called "multiomics" (Livingstone et al. 2015). The "omics" can be used to create personalized diagnostic and treatment procedures and increase their efficacy and safety. Precision medicine uses multiomic data to improve human health, better understand human biology, and create a perfect healthcare system that would be predictive, preventive, personalized, and participatory ("P4") (Ziegelstein 2017a; Guzzi et al. 2016). Most implementations of genomic profiling can be classified into one of two models based on the outcome: (1) research to discover generalized knowledge and (2) search to recover individualized knowledge (Trent 2019). A perfect example of therapy based on recovering individualized knowledge is chimeric antigen receptor T-cell therapy (CAR-T) using T cells grown in the laboratory to treat various types of cancer (Graham et al. 2018).

In the past, medicine has been practiced without evidence-based knowledge but medical care was adjusted to the individual. Current medicine has been dominated by technology, electronic documentation, and a race of time that often pulls the doctor away from the full care for patients. A question arises of effective doctor–patient communication. Ziegelstein (2017b) emphasizes that therapy, based on created guidelines, is tailored to groups rather than to individual patients, which makes the patient invisible in a group with similar diseases and characteristics. A new term has been adopted in clinical practice—"personomics"—to describe this unique phenomenon. Personalized medicine uses the knowledge about the patient's values, goals, preferences, and financial resources, all of which are included in "personomics". As Ziegelstein (2017b) states, "The evolution from precision medicine to personalized medicine is the evolution from healthcare to health caring". On the other hand, Jameson and Longo (2015) state that since medicine has been individualized and personalized, the term precision medicine should also consider the patient's psychosocial status. AI has strongly influenced personalized medicine. Consequently, the best possible solution for connecting personalized medicine with healthcare is to create a single process in which diagnosis, treatment, and follow-up of the patient are supplementary to each other and enable a fluent transition from one activity to another (Schork 2019). As the primary goal of precision medicine is developing models for humanity to predict the health status and prevent disease and disability, its application without using AI to process large data collection is next to impossible.

8 Artificial Intelligence (AI) in Medicine

The AI is tested in increasingly large medical fields. The first recognition came with the discovery that the computer-aided reading of mammograms is equal to the reading by a physician (Gilbert et al. 2008). Since that time, a lot of articles have described the application of AI in radiology and other fields of medical imaging, for example, pulmonology, invasive and noninvasive cardiology, psychiatry, or orthopedics (Kalmet et al. 2020; Refaee et al. 2020; Al'Aref et al. 2019; Davatzikos 2019; Betancur et al. 2018). Precision medicine offers a broad application of deep learning methods in defining features responsible for or predisposing to various diseases such as Alzheimer's, schizophrenia, dilated cardiomyopathy, or heart failure (Lin and Tsai 2019; Shah 2017). Genomic studies also amply use deep learning methods to name variants of protein sequences, predict mutation effects, or identify binding motifs (Bao et al. 2020). Of notable interest is a "deep patient" presented by Miotto et al. (2016), who have used the EHR to further clinical predictive modeling and observed substantial improvements in the diagnosis of testis and prostate cancers, sickle-cell anemia, attention deficit, and disruptive behavior disorders.

The proposed solutions influence the perception of modern medicine. The AI, whose increasing use is inescapable, substantially reduces healthcare costs. It helps doctors make their work and develop skills instead of spending time filling out medical records. The acceptance of AI in everyday life cannot adversely affect procedural outcomes and clinical efficacy. Conversely, it provides computational suggestions and models to avoid medical complications. The AI also makes it possible for doctors to extend the years of their active work time, with the accompanying advantages for the gross domestic product.

9 Conclusions

AI has undoubtedly improved medical care and management. Computer-based algorithms are time- and cost-effective measures that show the likely direction of future transformative developments (Anderson 2019). Innovative strategies in healthcare should center on the patient's well-being. Electronic health records help personalize medical care using technology as a consolidative tool. The AI is fundamental for the medical practice of excellence (Souza Filho et al. 2019). On the other side, there may be limitations for AI use in medicine. Some medical professionals harbor a bit of prejudice toward machine learning methods. Where the precision counts most, like in a healthcare system, there can be some selection pitfalls. The sampling and observer selection bias, indifferent in most commercial settings, can adversely affect the process of medical modeling. Selection bias can occur when an algorithm concludes deeply flawed data (Al'Aref et al. 2019). The occurrence of some diseases can be underpredicted due to inadequate screening, epidemiologic, or other poorly controlled factors. Such issues are difficult to identify and remedy in clinical trial datasets based on machine learning methods. Nonetheless, progress in the development of AI holds humanity's future in many a field, including resource efficiency, autonomous machines, healthcare, and the like. The AI is not likely to replace a man in many professions, but the expectation is that it will create more jobs than destroy, increasing productivity at the same time. As Ergen (2019) states, "The industrial era let machines do the physical work, the information era enabled machines to do the computation and storage, now the AI era will let machines make the decisions".

Conflicts of Interest The authors declare no conflicts of interest concerning this chapter.

Ethical Approval This chapter does not contain any studies with human participants or animals performed by any of the authors.

References

Agbo CC, Mahmoud QH, Eklund JM (2019) Blockchain technology in healthcare: a systematic review. Healthcare (Basel) 7(2):56

Aktolun C (2019) Artificial intelligence and radiomics in nuclear medicine: potentials and challenges. Eur J Nucl Med Mol Imaging 46(13):2731–2273

Al'Aref SJ, Anchouche K, Singh G, Slomka PJ, Kolli KK, Kumar A, Pandey M, Maliakal G, van Rosendael AR, Beecy AN, Berman DS, Leipsic J, Nieman K, Andreini D, Pontone G, Schoepf UJ, Shaw LJ, Chang HJ, Narula J, Bax JJ, Min JK (2019) Clinical applications of machine learning in cardiovascular disease and its relevance to cardiac imaging. Eur Heart J 40(24):1975–1986

Allam Z, Jones DS (2020) On the coronavirus (COVID-19) outbreak and the smart city network: universal data sharing standards coupled with artificial intelligence (AI) to benefit urban health monitoring and management. Healthcare (Basel) 8(1):46

Anderson KP (2019) Artificial intelligence-augmented ECG assessment: the promise and the challenge. J Cardiovasc Electrophysiol 30(5):675–678

Ash JS, Corby S, Mohan V, Solberg N, Becton J, Bergstrom R, Orwoll B, Hoekstra C, Gold JA (2020) Safe use of the EHR by medical scribes: a qualitative study. J Am Med Inform Assoc. https://doi.org/10.1093/jamia/ocaa199

Bao F, Deng Y, Du M, Ren Z, Wan S, Liang KY, Liu S, Wang B, Xin J, Chen F, Christiani DC, Wang M, Dai Q (2020) Explaining the genetic causality for complex phenotype via deep association kernel learning. Patterns (NY) 1(6):100057

Betancur J, Commandeur F, Motlagh M, Sharir T, Einstein AJ, Bokhari S, Fish MB, Ruddy TD, Kaufmann P, Sinusas AJ, Miller EJ, Bateman TM, Dorbala S, Di Carli M, Germano G, Otaki Y, Tamarappoo BK, Dey D, Berman DS, Slomka PJ (2018) Deep learning for prediction of obstructive disease from fast myocardial perfusion SPECT: a multicenter study. JACC Cardiovasc Imag 11(11):1654–1663

Bloom DE, Cadarette D (2019) Infectious disease threats in the twenty-first century: strengthening the global response. Front Immunol 10:549

Bush J, Baker S (2014) Where does it hurt? An entrepreneur's guide to fixing health care. Pengnin Group LLC, New York

Bycroft C, Freeman C, Petkova D, Band G, Elliott LT, Sharp K, Motyer A, Vukcevic D, Delaneau O, O'Connell J, Cortes A, Welsh S, Young A, Effingham M, McVean G, Leslie S, Allen N, Donnelly P, Marchini J (2018) The UK Biobank resource with deep phenotyping and genomic data. Nature 562(7726):203–209

Capolongo S, Rebecchi A, Buffoli M, Appolloni L, Signorelli C, Fara GM, D'Alessandro D (2020) COVID-19 and cities: from urban health strategies to the pandemic challenge. A decalogue of public health opportunities. Acta Biomed 91(2):13–22

Chen X, Dallmeier-Tiessen S, Dasler R (2019) Open is not enough. Nat Phys 15:113–119

Crampton NH, Reis S, Shachak A (2016) Computers in the clinical encounter: a scoping review and thematic analysis. J Am Med Inform Assoc 23(3):654–665

Dangelmeier W, Förster D, Hersthemke V, Kress S (1999) Survey of telework activities in Europe. In: Economic aspects of digital information technologies. Fachmedien. Springer, Wiesbaden

Davatzikos C (2019) Machine learning in neuroimaging: progress and challenges. NeuroImage 197:652–656

Deo RC (2015) Machine learning in medicine. Circulation 132(20):1920–1930

Eggebeen DJ, Lichter DT (1993) Health and well-being among rural Americans: variations across the life course. J Rural Health 9(2):86–98

Ergen M (2019) What is artificial intelligence? Technical considerations and future perception. Anatol J Cardiol 22(Suppl 2):5–7

Fore M (2019) With open data, scientists share their work. Symmetry Magazine. https://www.symmetrymagazine.org/article/with-open-data-scientists-share-their-work. Accessed 1 Dec 2020

Gawande A (2018) Why doctors hate their computers. Annals of Medicine. The New Yorker. https://www.newyorker.com/magazine/2018/11/12/why-doctors-hate-their-computers. Accessed 20 Nov 2020

Gilbert FJ, Astley SM, Gillan MG, Agbaje OF, Wallis MG, James J, Boggis CR, Duffy SW, CADET II Group (2008) Single reading with computer-aided detection for screening mammography. New Engl J Med 359(16):1675–1684

Global Liveability Index (2021) https://www.eiu.com/n/campaigns/global-liveability-index-2021/. Accessed 19 Oct 2021

Graham C, Jozwik A, Pepper A, Benjamin R (2018) Allogeneic CAR-T cells: more than ease of access? Cells 7 (10):155

Grzegorowska O, Lorkowski J (2020) Possible correlations between atherosclerosis, acute coronary syndromes and Covid-19. J Clin Med 9(11):3746

Guzzi PH, Agapito G, Milano M, Cannataro M (2016) Methodologies and experimental platforms for generating and analysing microarray and mass spectrometry-based omics data to support P4 medicine. Brief Bioinformatics 17(4):553–561

Haraldstad K, Wahl A, Andenæs R, Andersen JR, Andersen MH, Beisland E, Borge CR, Engebretsen E, Eisemann M, Halvorsrud L, Hanssen TA, Haugstvedt A, Haugland T, Johansen VA, Larsen MH, Løvereide L, Løyland B, Kvarme LG, Moons P, Norekvål TM, LIVSFORSK Network (2019) A systematic review of quality of life research in medicine and health sciences. Qual Life Res 28(10):2641–2650

Hawking S (2015) Reporting by Peter Vanham. Media Lead, US and Industries, Media Relations. World Economic Forum. https://www.weforum.org/agenda/2015/10/stephen-hawking-technology-seems-to-drive-ever-increasing-inequality/. Accessed 27 Nov 2020

Jameson JL, Longo DL (2015) Precision medicine – personalized, problematic, and promising. New Engl J Med 372(23):2229–2234

Juniper Research (2018). https://www.juniperresearch.com/harvest. Accessed 1 Jan 2021

Kalmet P, Sanduleanu S, Primakov S, Wu G, Jochems A, Refaee T, Ibrahim A, Hulst LV, Lambin P, Poeze M (2020) Deep learning in fracture detection: a narrative review. Acta Orthop 91(2):215–220

Kuo TT, Kim HE, Ohno-Machado L (2017) Blockchain distributed ledger technologies for biomedical and health care applications. J Am Med Inform Assoc 24 (6):1211–1220

Lewthwaite H, Effing TW, Olds T, Williams MT (2017) Physical activity, sedentary behaviour and sleep in COPD guidelines: a systematic review. Chronic Respir Dis 14(3):231–244

Lin S (2020) The present and future of team documentation: the role of patients, families, and artificial intelligence. Mayo Clin Proc 95(5):852–855

Lin E, Tsai SJ (2019) Machine learning in neural networks. Adv Exp Med Biol 1192:127–137

Livingstone SG, Smith MJ, Silva DS, Upshur RE (2015) Much ado about omics: welcome to 'the permutome'. J Eval Clin Pract 21(6):1018–1021

Lorkowski J, Malinowska M (2020) The future of medical documentation – review of selected literature. Preprints 2020050350. https://doi.org/10.20944/preprints202005.0350.v1

Marr B (2017) First FDA approval for clinical cloud-based deep learning in healthcare. In: Forbes. Forbes Publishing Company, New York City

Mearian L (2018) Amazon launches patient data-mining service to assist docs. Computerworld. https://www.computerworld.com/article/3324044/amazon-launchespatient-data-mining-service-to-assist-docs.html. Accessed 1 Dec 2020

Miotto R, Li L, Kidd BA, Dudley JT (2016) Deep patient: an unsupervised representation to predict the future of patients from the electronic health records. Sci Rep 6:26094

Park SH, Do KH, Kim S, Park JH, Lim YS (2019) What should medical students know about artificial intelligence in medicine? J Educ Eval Health Prof 16:18

Raulinajtys-Grzybek M, Lorkowski J (2020) How the organization of medical record keeping in a hospital ward affects the level of direct and indirect costs: model approach. Eurasian Studies in Business and Economics EJBE 17 (in press)

Refaee T, Wu G, Ibrahim A, Halilaj I, Leijenaar R, Rogers W, Gietema HA, Hendriks L, Lambin P, Woodruff HC (2020) The emerging role of radiomics in copd and lung cancer. Respiration 99(2):99–107

Riggs DW, Yeager RA, Bhatnagar A (2018) Defining the human envirome: an omics approach for assessing the environmental risk of cardiovascular disease. Circ Res 122(9):1259–1275

Sankar PL, Parker LS (2017) The precision medicine initiative's all of us research program: an agenda for research on its ethical, legal, and social issues. Genet Med 19(7):743–750

Schork NJ (2019) Artificial intelligence and personalized medicine. Cancer Treat Res 178:265–283

Seixas AA, Henclewood DA, Williams SK, Jagannathan R, Ramos A, Zizi F, Jean-Louis G (2018) Sleep duration and physical activity profiles associated with self-reported stroke in the United States: application of Bayesian belief network modeling techniques. Front Neurol 9:534

Shah SJ (2017) Precision medicine for heart failure with preserved ejection fraction: an overview. J Cardiovasc Transl Res 10(3):233–244

Smart Cities Association (2017). https://www.smartcitiesassociation.org/index.php/media-corner/news/164-singapore-tops-global-smart-city-performance-ranking-in-2017-study. Accessed 1 Jan 2017

Souza Filho EM, Fernandes FA, Soares C, Seixas FL, Santos A, Gismondi RA, Mesquita ET, Mesquita CT (2019) Artificial intelligence in cardiology: concepts, tools and challenges – "The horse is the one who runs, you must be the jockey". Arq Bras Cardiol 114 (4):718–725

Stouten P (2003) The new charter of Athens: towards sustainable neighbourhoods. Built Environ (1978–) 38(4):497–507

Toh CK, Sanguesa JA, Cano JC, Martinez FJ (2020) Advances in smart roads for future smart cities. Proc Math Phys Eng Sci 476(2233):20190439

Trent JM (2019) Foreword. Cancer Treat Res 178:v–vi

Winslow CE (1920) The untitled fields of public health. Science (NY) 51(1306):23–33

Zagozdzon P, Kolarzyk E, Marcinkowski JT (2011) Quality of life and rural place of residence in Polish women – population based study. AAEM 18(2):429–432

Ziegelstein RC (2017a) Personomics: the missing link in the evolution from precision medicine to personalized medicine. J Pers Med 7(4):11

Ziegelstein RC (2017b) Personomics and precision medicine. Trans Am Clin Climatol Assoc 128:160–168

Adv Exp Med Biol - Clinical and Experimental Biomedicine (2022) 13: 11–35
https://doi.org/10.1007/5584_2021_626

Published online: 2 March 2021

Complex Interaction Among Immune, Inflammatory, and Carcinogenic Mechanisms in the Head and Neck Squamous Cell Carcinoma

Ana Caruntu, Cristian Scheau, Mircea Tampa, Simona Roxana Georgescu, Constantin Caruntu, and Cristiana Tanase

Abstract

Inflammation is deeply involved in the development of most types of cancer. Many studies focus on the interaction between immune-inflammatory mechanisms and tumorigenesis in the head and neck squamous cell carcinoma (HNSCC). In this chapter, we emphasize the complexity of processes underlying this interaction and discuss the mechanisms of carcinogenesis in HNSCC with a special focus on metabolic changes, inflammation, and the immune landscape. Unveiling complex connections between immuno-inflammatory processes and tumor initiation, promotion, and progression will open new directions in the reliable identification of predictive factors and therapeutic targets in HNSCC.

A. Caruntu
Department of Oral and Maxillofacial Surgery, "Carol Davila" Central Military Emergency Hospital, Bucharest, Romania

Faculty of Dental Medicine, "Titu Maiorescu" University, Bucharest, Romania
e-mail: ana.caruntu@gmail.com

C. Scheau
Department of Physiology, "Carol Davila" University of Medicine and Pharmacy, Bucharest, Romania
e-mail: cristian.scheau@umfcd.ro

M. Tampa (✉) and S. R. Georgescu
Department of Dermatology, "Victor Babes" Clinical Hospital for Infectious Diseases, Bucharest, Romania

Department of Dermatology, "Carol Davila" University of Medicine and Pharmacy, Bucharest, Romania
e-mail: tampa_mircea@yahoo.com; simonaroxanageorgescu@yahoo.com

C. Caruntu (✉)
Department of Physiology, "Carol Davila" University of Medicine and Pharmacy, Bucharest, Romania

Department of Dermatology, "Prof. N.C. Paulescu" National Institute of Diabetes, Nutrition, and Metabolic Diseases, Bucharest, Romania
e-mail: costin.caruntu@gmail.com

C. Tanase
Faculty of Dental Medicine, "Titu Maiorescu" University, Bucharest, Romania

Department of Biochemistry-Proteomics, "Victor Babes" National Institute of Pathology, Bucharest, Romania
e-mail: cristianatp@yahoo.com

Keywords

Cancer · Head and neck squamous cell carcinoma · Immunity · Inflammation · Therapy · Tumorigenesis

1 Introduction

Inflammation is deeply involved in the development and progression of most cancers, even if, at first glance, the mechanisms of inflammation are not prominent actors (Taniguchi and Karin 2018). Inflammation has been recognized as a promoter at all stages of tumorigenesis (Greten and Grivennikov 2019). Hence, it is not surprising that researchers have focused on studying the relations between immune-inflammatory mechanisms and tumorigenesis in different types of cancer, including head and neck squamous altering the cell carcinoma (HNSCC) (Georgescu et al. 2020; Scheau et al. 2020; Neagu et al. 2019; Tampa et al. 2018a; Tampa et al. 2018b; Georgescu et al. 2017; Neagu et al. 2016).

HNSCC is the world's sixth most frequent cancer, with an increasing incidence during the last decades, as life expectancy and global population increase (Economopoulou and Psyrri 2017). Despite great progress in diagnosing and treating cancers, death rates associated with HNSCC did not decrease significantly, due most likely to a high rate of the first diagnosis in advanced stages of the disease (Jou and Hess 2017). When early diagnosed and treated, survival rates in patients with HNSCC exceed 80–90% (NIH 2017). When distant metastases occur, although rare compared to other cancers, a high death toll of 74% at 24 months is present (Wiegand et al. 2015). This condition is commonly diagnosed in adult and elderly population, but recent data show a decreasing trend of the onset age. Men are three times more likely to develop HNSCC, but lately, an increasing incidence has also been reported in women (Chi et al. 2015).

2 Etiopathogenic Features of HNSCC in Different Locations

HNSCC includes a series of malignancies with different anatomical locations, for example, lip, oral, sinus cavities, pharynx and larynx, which are grouped according to etiopathogenic similarities, as well as clinical, therapeutic, and evolution criteria (Faraji et al. 2017).

Various endogenous and environmental factors participate in the development and progression of regional HNSCC (Solomon et al. 2018; Wu et al. 2018; Lupu et al. 2017; Voiculescu et al. 2016). For example, ultraviolet (UV) radiation is the main risk factor for lip and skin SCC as damaged. Keratinocytes accumulate mutations (Lupu et al. 2020; Chan et al. 2019; Lupu et al. 2018a, b). The UV exposure is also associated with the release of pro-inflammatory cytokines, such as TNF-α, stimulating the differentiation of monocytes into macrophages and maintaining local inflammation, which may induce angiogenesis and tumor progression (Bottomley et al. 2019). Moreover, inhibition of antitumor response in CD4+ and CD8+ lymphocytes against keratinocytes with alterations induced by UV radiation has been reported (Suwanpradid et al. 2017). Exposure to UV radiation has also been investigated in the context of decreasing density of the antigen-presenting. Langerhans and dendritic epidermis-resident cells. The apoptosis of these cells may exert Th2 and Treg-related immunosuppressive effects altering the antitumor immune response (Otsuka et al. 2018; Pettersen et al. 2011).

In HNSCC, smoking and chronic alcohol consumption are involved in more than 75% of cases (Hashibe et al. 2007). When these factors are combined, their damaging effects are enhanced and the risk of developing HNSCC can increase by 35-fold (Economopoulou and Psyrri 2017). Tobacco use induces epigenetic alterations in oral mucosa, with modified expression of various genes such as p53, GLUT-1, p16, and P13K in oral epithelial cells. It can impair various immune mechanisms involved in antitumor response and can activate oxidative stress reactions, leading to increased expression of pro-inflammatory genes and status of chronic inflammation (Jiang et al. 2019; Khowal and Wajid 2019; Seifi et al. 2014). Alcohol increases the permeability of oral mucosa for carcinogens. It also generates toxic compounds that can induce DNA damage and stimulate cell proliferation. Chronic alcohol intake is also associated with free radicals production that may induce immunosuppression (Feller et al. 2013).

Human papillomavirus (HPV) infection is mainly associated with oropharyngeal cancers, exhibiting a different behavior compared to tobacco- and alcohol-induced cancers (Tampa et al. 2020; Boda et al. 2018; Georgescu et al. 2018; Kobayashi et al. 2018; Boda et al. 2016). Almost half of these carcinomas are correlated with an active HPV status (Quabius et al. 2015). The most prevalent viral types are HPV16, HPV18, and HPV33 (Faraji et al. 2017; Ndiaye et al. 2014). Studies on a large number of patients have suggested that HPV+ tumors should be considered as distinct pathological entities within the wide group of HNSCC due to specific molecular features that correlate with improved response to therapy and prognosis (Dayyani et al. 2010). The 2017 classification of the tumor (T), nodes (N), and metastases (M) (TNM) has been updated according to these findings (Amin et al. 2017). Moreover, individualized therapies are proposed based on the HPV status (Cao et al. 2017; Husain and Neyaz 2017; Keck et al. 2015). There is a complex connection between HPV infection and chronic inflammation as the inflammatory cytokines can facilitate viral penetration and survival in the oral mucosa. They can also influence the proliferation of keratinocytes and viral activation (Tezal 2012; Tezal et al. 2012). Other studies have shown that HPV infection is associated with an increased T-cell infiltration and immune cell activation, considering the HPV status as a predictive factor for programmed cell death protein 1 (PD-1) inhibitors' therapeutic efficacy in HNSCC (Wang et al. 2019; Gameiro et al. 2018).

Occupational exposure to carcinogens like wood, textiles, or leather compounds is incriminated in the development of sino-nasal SCC. These tumors have a poor prognosis, especially when correlated with smoking, considering that most patients show advanced disease staging at the time of diagnosis (Elgart and Faden 2020).

A glance at the main risk factors of HNSCC and their mechanisms of action brings to attention the interconnections between inflammation, immune factors, and carcinogenic processes (see Fig. 1). To unravel the complexity of these processes, in the following sections we delineate the mechanisms of carcinogenesis in HNSCC with a special focus on metabolic changes, inflammation, and the immune landscape. We also highlight the importance of this topic for the discovery of new biomarkers and emerging therapies for HNSCC.

3 Mechanisms of Carcinogenesis in HNSCC

3.1 Genetic Traits in HNSCC

The mechanism of cancer initiation has been intensely studied over the years. The first step in the understanding of carcinogenesis was Rudolf Virchow's description of cancer cells (see McManus 1958). Shortly afterward, Theodor Boveri described the uncontrolled division of cells with a modified nuclear content in cancers, and these changes were linked to external factors (see Opitz 2016). Decades later, the first oncogene v-Src and the first tumor suppressor gene (TSG) were discovered, confirming the genetic basis of carcinogenesis (Alfred and Knudson 1971; Duesberg and Vogt 1970). Experimental murine models have been created through genetic engineering over the last years, with the intent of studying various types of cancer (Kersten et al. 2017). DNA sequencing techniques have revolutionized medical research allowing the characterization of the entire genome, including the mutations that trigger tumors (International Human Genome Sequencing Consortium 2004). Focal mutations, deletions, duplications, or

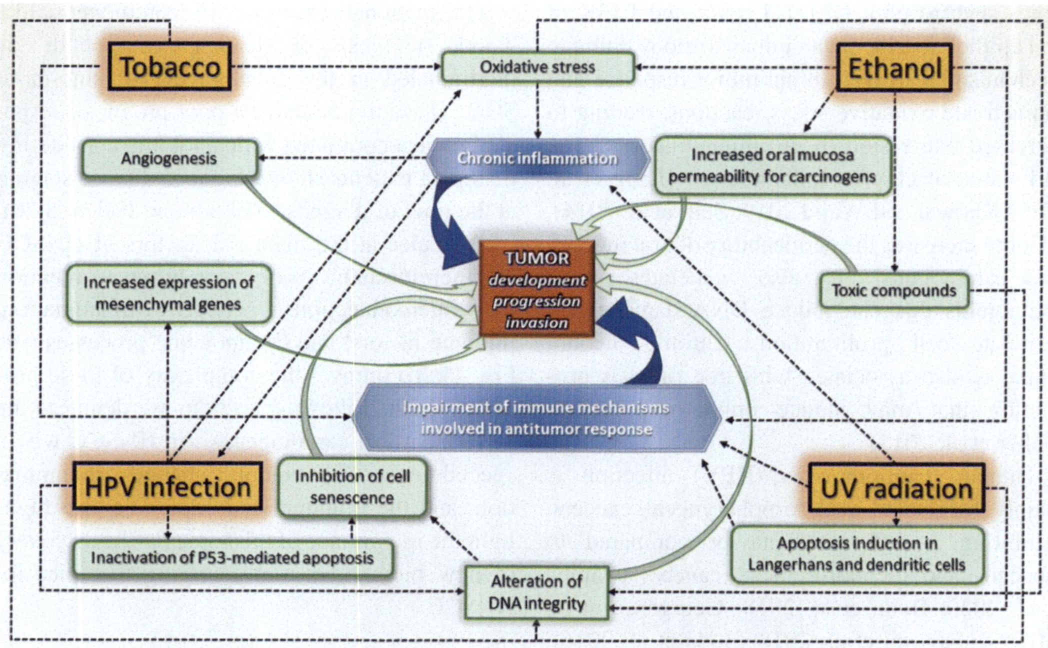

Fig. 1 Interconnections between inflammation, immune factors, and carcinogenic processes associated with the main risk factors of head and neck squamous cell carcinoma (HNSCC)

insertions of nucleotides contribute to the tumor mutational burden (TMB). A genetic database analysis has identified patterns of mutated genes, attributing genetic signatures to each type of neoplasia (Fancello et al. 2019; Chalmers et al. 2017).

HNSCC arises frequently from premalignant lesions, with a gradual accumulation of mutations associated with long-time exposure to external carcinogens in addition to increased age-related DNA instability (Monisha et al. 2017). Mutations of the tumor suppressor TP53 gene have been identified in most cancers (Perri et al. 2016) and in more than 70% of HNSCC (Pérez Sayáns et al. 2019). Labeled "guardian of the genome", the TP53 acts through multiple intracellular signaling pathways controlling processes like DNA repair, cell cycle arrest, and apoptosis. A transition to altered phenotype induces resistance to apoptosis, genome instability, and decreased immunogenicity (Perdrix et al. 2017). In nicotine-induced HNSCC, TP53 mutations with loss of function are almost constantly present (Cancer Genome Atlas Network 2015), even from very early stages, affecting guanosine nucleotides (Denaro et al. 2011). Deletions in the tumor-suppressing CDKN2A gene are in the top five most frequent mutations in the smoking-induced HNSCC. When associated, mutations in CDKN2A and TP53 genes negatively impact survival (Pérez Sayáns et al. 2019).

In contrast, HPV-positive tumors exhibit a low mutational burden involving these two suppressor genes. The overexpression of specific viral HPV E6/7genes, amplification of PIK3CA and E2F1 genes, and a loss of TRAF3 are the most representative genetic changes (Cancer Genome Atlas Network 2015). HPV infection, acting through viral oncoproteins E6 and E7, inactivates tumor supressor genes pRb and p53 in the host cell, leading to a loss of cell-cycle control, chromosomal instability, impaired DNA repair, and alterations in cell senescence and apoptosis (Castellanos and Pan 2016; Kim 2016; Doorbar et al. 2015). The recent research has broadened the spectrum of effects induced by HPV infection, showing that the E6 oncoprotein increases the levels of reactive oxygen species and oxidative stress. This effect increases DNA instability and may be associated with chronic inflammation (Cruz-Gregorio et al. 2019).

Other studies have reported alterations in several representatives of the "rat sarcoma" (RAS) oncogene family in HNSCC. The HRAS isoform is mutated in 6% of HNSCC and associated with enhanced immune activity, with a high density of immune effectors in tumor samples (Lyu et al. 2019). The KRAS isoform is isolated in 17% of patients with HNSCC and associated with altered immune mechanisms, promoting immune tolerance via transforming growth factor-beta 1 (TGF-β1) (Weidhaas et al. 2017; Calenic et al. 2015).

Other genetic changes are independent of the HPV status. The activation of nuclear factor kappa-light-chain-enhancer of activated B cells (NF-κB), consequent to a loss of TP53, exerts pro-carcinogenetic effects by stimulating cell proliferation, angiogenesis, and epithelial to mesenchymal transition (EMT) (Aggarwal et al. 2006; Bharti and Aggarwal 2002). Experimental studies on HNSCC have revealed that a high intracellular concentration of active NF-κB is associated with increased metastatic capacity. NF-κB inhibitors are successful in decreasing cell invasive features by decreasing enzymes related to metastasis, such as vascular endothelial growth factor (VEGF) and matrix metallopeptidase 9 (MMP-9) (Yan et al. 2010). The activation of NF-κB has been detected in precancerous lesions frequently associated with HNSCC and in radio- and chemoresistant diseases. Deactivation of NF-κB in tumor cells leads to tumor regression in experimental models, triggering great interest in cancer therapy development.

While mandatory, genetic mutations are insufficient to develop cancer. The malignant cell requires appropriate conditions to multiply in an environment that provides protection from systemic tumor clearance mechanisms (Wellenstein and de Visser 2018).

3.2 Metabolic Changes in HNSCC

Frequent mitoses, characteristic of malignant cells, require high energy resources, implying an increased intracellular metabolism to cover the energy demand. Intense metabolic activity increases oxygen requirements, and tumor cells shift towards glycolysis to supplement energy production, leading to a decreased intracellular pH and accumulation of acidic byproducts. Intracellular acidosis seems an important element in local tumor progression and metastasis (Hosseini et al. 2017). Acidic pH of 6.5–6.9 is detected in the peritumoral environment. The theory of "acid-mediated tumor invasion" claims that a peritumoral acidic environment triggers necrosis in normal cells through pH-induced metabolic changes and activates MMPs that degrade the extracellular matrix, facilitating metastasis. Local acidosis exerts inhibitory effects on antitumoral immunity, promoting tumor progression. Various cancer experimental models show significant expression of markers for acidosis LAMP (lysosomal-associated membrane protein) and hypoxia (glucose transporter 1 and carbonic anhydrase IX (CA-IX)) (Ibrahim-Hashim and Estrella 2019). The CO_2 produced in tumoral metabolic conditions is eliminated from the cell via CA-IX activity, a membrane transporter that hydrates CO_2 and exports it as HCO_3^- and H^+ (Tafreshi et al. 2014). CA-IX activity is accelerated at pKa values under 6.5, modulating the acidity of a peritumoral environment. The inhibition of antitumoral immune surveillance is another consequence of acidosis, with alterations in cytolytic functions, a reduction of cytokine secretion, and the inhibition of signal transducers and activators of transcription 5/extracellular signal-regulated kinases (STAT5/ERK) signaling pathway (Calcinotto et al. 2012). In vivo experiments demonstrate that the use of oral buffer products correlates with increased efficiency of monoclonal antibody-based therapies (Pilon-Thomas et al. 2016).

Oxidative stress is closely correlated with carcinogenesis. Malignant cells show increased production of reactive oxygen species (ROS) induced by exogenous or endogenous stimuli. ROS promote carcinogenesis through DNA instability. The subsequent mechanisms are tyrosine phosphatase inactivation and activation of the hypoxia-inducible factor 1 alpha (HIF-1α) pathway, which sustains malignant cell proliferation and immune cell anergy by further shifting cell metabolism to glycolysis (Vomund et al. 2017). In head and neck cancers, exposures to antioxidative agents, glutathione, and thioredoxin exert a strong inhibitory effect on cell proliferation and tumor growth (Roh et al. 2017). Multiple genetic alterations and metabolic changes are associated with tumor growth and metastasis in HNSCC. The effervescence of intracellular and local carcinogenic events generates a systemic response to counterbalance the progression to malignancy.

3.3 Inflammation in HNSCC

Chronic inflammation is an important element in carcinogenesis. Numerous studies show that indices of inflammation, assessed in the tumor tissue or peripheral blood, correlate with patient survival and response to therapy, leading to the evaluation of different inflammatory factors as biomarkers in HNSCC (Tampa et al. 2018b). Cytokines are small proteins released mainly by T helper cells and macrophages that play an essential role in regulating the immune response. Even though the immune cells are the primary source of cytokines, any nucleated cell carries the enzymes required for the synthesis and release of cytokines (Zhang and An 2007; Dinarello 2000). Pro-inflammatory interleukins have been intensively studied in the pathogenesis of HNSCC. The tumor milieu is characterized by chronic inflammation induced by various cellular and humoral mediated processes involving tumor, stromal, and immune cells. Increased concentrations of pro-inflammatory chemokines are reported in association with an inflammatory infiltration rich in macrophages, fibroblasts, and monocytes. Wang et al. (2002) have analyzed 86 tissue samples of HNSCC and demonstrated the overexpression of interleukin 6 (IL-6) and IL-6 messenger RNA compared to normal mucosa. This study also reveals a correlation between receptor expression for IL-6 and the tumor size and grading. IL-6 mRNA overexpression is associated with advanced disease and lymph and distant metastases. A study that assessed the immune gene expression in advanced HNSCC defined two out of the four tumor types with distinct immune profiles, presumably correlating with the HPV status. Pro-inflammatory cytokines and immune cell effectors were at high concentrations in the tumor microenvironment, defined as an enriched immune microenvironment (EIME), and correlated with prognosis (Cao et al. 2017). Sato et al. (2013) have suggested that determining salivary levels of IL-6 after treatment could act as a biomarker for early local and regional recurrence in HNSCC, while Jinno et al. (2015) have argued that IL-6 overexpression is associated with chemoresistant disease.

Significant correlations are also reported between cytokine levels and the progression of premalignant lesions to invasive malignant disease. Schiegnitz et al. (2018) have identified increased serum concentrations of IL-6, IL-8, and soluble IL-2 receptors in patients with HNSCC compared to patients who are either healthy or suffer from premalignant conditions, with IL-6 demonstrating a high statistical significance with large tumors and lymph node metastasis. The same study reports that patients with premalignant lesions have higher levels of IL-8 than controls. Salivary levels of IL-8 have been analyzed in patients suffering from premalignant lesions and oral squamous cell carcinoma compared to healthy subjects. The results demonstrate that only subjects with invasive lesions show significantly higher concentrations of IL-8, thus recommending salivary IL-8 as a potential biomarker for the diagnosis and follow-up of oral squamous cell carcinoma, but not of premalignant lesions (Punyani and Sathawane 2013). The NF-κB pathway discussed above might be the underlying mechanism for IL-8-mediated HNSCC tumorigenesis, confirming the role of chronic inflammation in malignant transformation (Rao et al. 2010).

Interactions between inflammation and carcinogenesis described in oral squamous cell carcinoma have also been identified in cutaneous squamous cell carcinoma (Scheau et al. 2020). In UV-induced skin and lip cancers, activation of intracellular NF-κB signaling pathways triggers a cascade of inflammatory events, including the secretion of IL-8 by macrophages and monocytes, which eventually leads to tumor progression (Neagu et al. 2019; Balkwill and Coussens 2004). The involvement of chronic inflammation, fueled by the release of cytokines, underlies malignant transformation, local invasion, and metastases. Conversely, inhibition of the immune response by anti-inflammatory agents correlates with a decrease in UV-induced cancer incidence (Wright et al. 2006).

The anti-inflammatory cytokines IL-10 and IL-13 have been found significantly increased in saliva of HNSCC patients and tumor tissue of oral squamous cell carcinoma (Aziz et al. 2015; Chen et al. 2013). The increase correlates with poor prognosis, especially in early disease, suggesting that a strong immunosuppressive environment at the initial stages is conducive to aggressive tumor cell behavior, promoting tumor growth and progression.

3.4 Assessment of Inflammation in HNSCC in Clinical Setting

The detection of sophisticated elements for cancer diagnosis in early stages and disease follow-up requires expensive laboratory equipment, trained staff, expensive kits, which may be available in a research unit, but are difficult to access in the clinical setting for general use. The current clinical practice evaluates inflammation through cellular and biochemical markers of the systemic immune response, and several studies have reported results that support the prognostic value of markers in various cancers.

Circulating proteins involved in systemic inflammation have been studied as potential prognostic biomarkers in different malignancies. C reactive protein (CRP) increases in inflammation, infection, and trauma. Recent data show a strong correlation between the CRP level and cancer. A study that followed a large group of subjects from the general population for 16 years has reported an increased rate of malignancies in patients with a high serum CRP content. Additionally, increased baseline CRP in cancer patients was associated with poor prognosis (Allin et al. 2009). The onset of cancer correlates with sustained inflammatory status induced by the intense metabolic reactions in tumor tissue. This systemic inflammatory process, translated in increased serum content of CRP, among other changes, is described in cancer patients (Asegaonkar et al. 2015). In OSCC, higher values of CRP are detected in patients exposed to risk factors (smoking and alcohol) and correlate with an increased rate of regional progression through lymph node involvement and poor prognosis (Tai et al. 2017). Similar results in HNSCC are reported in several studies, correlating an aggressive tumor behavior with unfavorable prognosis and elevated levels of CRP (Peter et al. 2013; Khandavilli et al. 2009). Some authors studied CRP in relation to other parameters. Glasgow prognostic score and its refined variants include serum albumin, alongside CRP, and are used in stratifying the clinical risk of patients with various cancers (Pan et al. 2017; Saijo et al. 2017). These scores have been analyzed in patients with operable HNSCC and reported data to support their prognostic potential (Hanai et al. 2018; Selzer et al. 2016; Farhan-Alanie et al. 2015).

Serum fibrinogen correlates with disease progression in different cancers (Zhang et al. 2020; Xu et al. 2018). This glycoprotein, known for its role in coagulation, is also involved in the cancer-associated systemic inflammatory response, and elevated levels of fibrinogen correlate with poor prognosis in many malignancies (Grafetstätter et al. 2019). In solid tumors, progression to malignancy and local invasiveness correlate with changes in structural components present in the extracellular environment. Deposits of fibrinogen and fibrin have been identified in tumor stroma promoting fibroblast proliferation and angiogenesis mediated by overexpression of IL-1, VEGF (vascular endothelial growth factor), and FGF-2 (fibroblast growth factor 2) (Mosesson 2005;

Simpson-Haidaris and Rybarczyk 2001). The link between fibrinogen and cancer progression is still unclear. However, various studies reveal strong correlations with prognosis in patients with HNSCC. In locally advanced OSCC, high pretreatment fibrinogen values have been detected in patients with resistance to radio- and chemotherapy and correlated with disease recurrence and poor survival (Holzinger et al. 2016). Other studies have shown similar results in HNSCC, where a high serum fibrinogen content correlates with advanced disease, presence of metastases, and unfavorable prognosis (Yang et al. 2019; Lan et al. 2016).

4 Immune Landscape in Carcinogenesis

4.1 Defensive Mechanisms Against Cancer

The role of the immune system in carcinogenesis was suspected more than a century ago by W.B. Coley, a surgeon who reported a series of cases treated by bacterial inoculation in tumor mass. The therapy relied on triggering a local immune response that would destroy tumor cells (Coley 1910). The important role of the immune system in the protection against cancer was confirmed by the substantial increase in the incidence of cancers, especially viral related, in subjects with immunodeficiency syndromes of various causes (Vajdic and Van Leeuwen 2009).

In the complex antitumor defense machinery, intrinsic cellular mechanisms are doubled by extrinsic protection systems in which immune cells are key players. While intrinsic tumor suppression mechanisms are active and efficient, the immune response is not initiated. The accumulation of genetic alterations, such as mutations of the p53 suppressor gene, leads to an increased intracellular concentration of p53 peptide, shifting the metabolic pattern of the affected cell. Subsequently, opposing intracellular mechanisms are overcome and the mutant cell is beyond repair, entering a stabilization phase called cellular senescence, which implies changes in its secretory phenotype (Kuilman et al. 2010). It initiates the release of pro-inflammatory cytokines generating an immune reaction guided to destroy the senescent cell, thus preventing the progression to malignancy (Kuilman et al. 2008). An increased density of cells with the senescence-associated secretory phenotype (SASP) is reported in precancerous lesions of OSCC, which may act as the first step in cancer prevention by inducing a lymphocyte T CD4+ mediated immune response (Johnson et al. 2016; Campo-Trapero et al. 2008). Progressive mutations with p53 loss of function together with other gene alterations push mutant cells out of SASP status leading to the development of invasive features (Wellenstein and de Visser 2018). In this stage of carcinogenesis, if the balance favors the accumulation of mutations and overruns the clearance capacity of the immune system, malignant cells survive, setting the debut of cancer. In established malignancies, lymphocytes T CD8+ are the main antitumor effectors. Little mobilization of these cells in premalignant lesions could be a prevention mechanism of autoimmunity mediated by cytotoxic T lymphocytes (Ostroumov et al. 2018). Studies conducted on murine models show that CD4+ T lymphocytes that release interferon-gamma (IFN-γ) and TNF-α can reactivate the SASP mechanisms and induce growth arrest in tumor cells, promoting immune clearance of malignant cells, independently from intracellular protection mechanisms (Braumüller et al. 2013).

Three steps have been defined in the immune antitumor defense process: elimination, equilibrium, and escape (see Fig. 2). Throughout these steps, immune cells undergo tumor immunoediting, a process in which highly immunogenic cells with an intense expression of tumor-specific antigens (TSA) are removed. In the experimental setting, tumor cells generated in immunodeficient animal models do not progress to malignancy after transplantation into immunocompetent hosts, because the immunoediting and proliferation of poorly immunogenic cell lines do not take place (Smyth et al. 2006). In the initial elimination phase, newly created tumor cells are efficiently removed by the immune system (Mittal

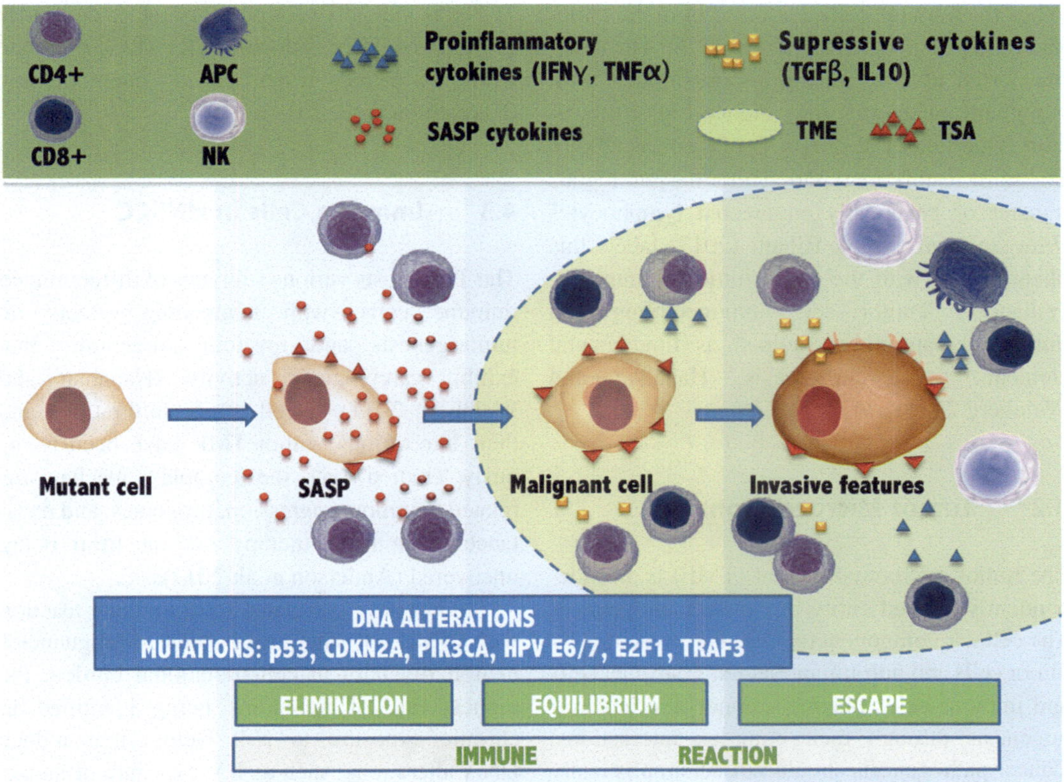

Fig. 2 Graphic representation of genetic and immune dysfunctions leading to carcinogenesis. Progressive accumulation of intracellular genetic alterations leads to a switch to senescence-associated secretory phenotype (SASP) with specific cytokine release that initiates activation of the immune response, mainly mediated by CD4+ lymphocytes. Intensely immunogenic cells, expressing tumor-specific antigens (TSA) are eliminated, leading to the selection of mutant clones with decreased immunogenicity in the equilibrium phase. Tumor microenvironment (TME) formation is initiated with modulatory effects on immune effectors promoting progression to cancer with invasive features. In the escape phase, progressive accumulation of immune cells: CD8+ lymphocytes, natural killer cells (NK), antigen-presenting cells (APC) together with CD4+ lymphocytes can be detected, with different, often antagonistic, effects on tumor growth

et al. 2014). This may explain the spontaneous tumor remission described in clinically manifest malignancies (Markowska and Markowska 1998). Overcoming the capacity of immune clearance of malignant cells pushes forward carcinogenesis into the equilibrium phase, where tumor progression is controlled by immune surveillance mechanisms. Malignant cells will not be fully eliminated, and by adding new mutations, they will generate cellular clones with decreased immunogenicity. The tumor microenvironment is initiated in this stage of carcinogenesis, which will promote survival of malignant cells and finally advancement to the escape phase of the immune response, favoring cancer progression (Bottomley et al. 2019). Equilibrium phase mechanisms might explain the pathogenesis of occult malignancies, frequently encountered in HNSCC, where the immune system counteracts local tumor development (Koebel et al. 2007). The clinical manifestation of cancer occurs when tumor cells have survived the intrinsic antitumor control mechanisms, the senescent cell elimination phase, and have passed immunoediting processes. However, tumor cells never achieve a complete immunotolerance state.

When the immune cells, collected from the tumor microenvironment and processed in vitro, are transferred to lymphopenic mouse models with malignant melanoma, they induce tumor regression (Quezada et al. 2010; Dudley et al. 2008). The same results are reported after the autologous transfer of genetically engineered lymphocytes (Morgan et al. 2006). Ribatti (2017) labels this phenomenon with the term "tumor immunosurveillance". Tumor cell immunoediting and immune escaping are defined as fundamental elements of carcinogenesis (Hanahan and Weinberg 2011).

4.2 Tumor Microenvironment

The tumor microenvironment (TME) is an independently studied entity in cancer pathogenesis. The cellular component in TME is represented by tumor cells and non-tumor elements: stromal cells and immune cells, playing a major role in carcinogenesis through their complex interactions. Cancer pathogenesis should not be simplistically regarded as a sum of tumor cell features but rather as a distinct structure with independent pathophysiological characteristics. Inflammatory tumor infiltrations are present in all cancers, with variable intensity, ranging from patterns undetectable through standard evaluation techniques to intense inflammatory types of cancer. The complex interactions between stromal components of TME, inflammatory, and tumor cells are not yet completely unveiled (Thorsson et al. 2018; Cai and Jin 2017).

Tumor stromal acellular composition can vary from a high content of loose connective tissue to an increased number of collagen structures that grant a fibrotic aspect to the lesion. These stromal elements can organize tumor cell nests (TCN) of variable size, with presumed prognostic characteristics in several malignancies (Alsibai and Meseure 2018; van Pelt et al. 2018). A recent study has analyzed several specific tumor stroma parameters, such as stroma-tumor ratio (TSR), stroma type, and TCN size in patients with HNSCC, showing that the increased TSR, defined by a fibrotic stroma with frequent small-sized TCNs, is indicative for poor prognosis contrarily to the large TCN and low TSR, which correlate with a better response to chemotherapy (Karpathiou et al. 2019).

4.3 Immune Cells in HNSCC

The TME hosts various subtypes of differentiated immune cells, with contrasting effects on tumorigenesis and myeloid progenitors that exhibit carcinogenic activity (Hanahan and Weinberg 2011). T-cell tumor infiltrations and their interactions within TME have been rigorously studied, yet the complex mechanisms related to tumor progression, prognosis, and resistance to immune therapy are far from being uncovered (Anderson et al. 2017).

Studies have correlated local immune reaction with TMB of malignant cells. Malignancies exhibit diversity in cell mutational burden, the highest rate of mutations being identified in chronic exposure to risk factors that induce DNA alterations, such as UV exposure or smoking. In consequence, UV and nicotine-induced squamous cell carcinomas have been reported to possess one of the highest mutational burdens (Fancello et al. 2019). Tumors with a high TMB are characterized by an increased expression of tumor-specific antigens (Rooney et al. 2015). These antigens result from degrading self-proteins into 8–10 amino acid-long peptides that activate T-cells, triggering an antitumor immune reaction (Antunes et al. 2018). Both innate and adaptive immune systems are directed towards eliminating malignant cells, through mechanisms mediated by major histocompatibility complex (MHC), implying TSA-mediated activation of immune effectors. Except for viral-induced malignancies (HPV or EBV), tumor cells derived from self-structures expressing MHC Class I should not trigger an immune response. However, TSAs are presented mainly through MHC class I and can be recognized by the immune effectors (Schumacher et al. 2019). Decreased expression of MHC Class I molecules on tumor cells is another mechanism of immune escape. However, malignant cells with negative MHC Class I status are eliminated by NK cells (Garrido 2019). NK cells show an increased affinity for cancers with low or lacking MHC Class I expression, called "missing self" cells, by recognizing the absence of normal elements on the cell surface known as "absence of the expected" (Kärre 2008). This phenomenon is used on developing molecules that promote NK-mediated tumor cell clearance, either independently or in association with T lymphocytes, especially in MHC Class I-negative cancers (Minetto et al. 2019). In HPV-positive HNSCC, MHC Class II plays an important role. Viral antigens bind to MHC Class II molecules that are overexpressed on tumor cells, acting as antigen-presenting cells. An intense immune response is generated that is associated with a significantly improved prognosis (Gameiro et al. 2019). However, overexpression of TSAs is present only on a subpopulation of tumor cells, triggering an ineffective immune response that may explain resistance to targeted therapies (McGranahan et al. 2016). Based on these findings, some cancers, including HNSCC, are divided into subtypes according to immune and genetic features that correlate with prognosis and response to therapy (Cao et al. 2017; Keck et al. 2015).

Tumor-infiltrating lymphocytes (TILs) show high variability in cancers. Cytotoxic T-cells (CD8+), helper T-cells (CD4+), regulatory T-cells (Treg), and B lymphocytes coexist in TME with the leucocytes of the innate immune family, such as NK cells, innate lymphoid cells (ILC), macrophages, neutrophils, monocytes, antigen-presenting cells (APC), and dendritic cells, exerting synergic or antagonistic effects.

Cytotoxic T-Cells (CD8+) The main effectors of adaptive immune responses, when present in large numbers in TME, predict a better prognosis in most cancers (Mazzaschi et al. 2018; Li et al. 2017). Similar results have been reported for patients with HNSCC, where the density and distribution of CD8+ lymphocytes in TME seem to have independent prognostic capabilities (see Table 1). A study conducted on 139 patients with oral squamous cell carcinoma has reported that high numbers of CD8+ T-cells in parenchyma around the invasion front and stromal CD8+ cells at the tumor periphery independently correlated with improved survival and low recurrence rates (Shimizu et al. 2019). HPV status in HNSCC plays an important role in the immune infiltration of TME. Thus, HPV-positive tumors show a higher CD8+ T-cell infiltration compared to HPV-negative ones in oropharyngeal squamous cell carcinoma, which also correlates with better prognosis when CD8+ T-cells concentrate in stromal areas (Oguejiofor et al. 2015). This finding most likely relies on the synergic immune recruitment mechanisms mediated by two distinct triggers, TSA and viral antigens, which intensify the local immune reactivity. Näsman et al. (2012) have reported similar results in tonsillar SCC in that patients with HPV-positive tumors display a higher number of CD8+ T-cells compared to HPV-negative ones, and an enriched CD8+ T-cell environment correlates with better survival. Another study conducted on 270 subjects with oropharyngeal squamous cell carcinoma has identified a small subgroup of patients with HPV-positive tumors that exhibited low concentrations of tumor-infiltrating lymphocytes (TILs), with a prognosis similar to HPV-negative tumors (Ward et al. 2014). CD8+ T-cells rely on interaction with CD4+ T lymphocytes to exert their cytotoxic functions.

Helper T Lymphocytes (CD4+) They initiate and maintain antitumor immune reaction by mobilizing CD8+ T-cells that recognize specific tumor antigens presented by MHC molecules and trigger tumor cell death (Ostroumov et al. 2018). T helper cells are involved in all aspects of antitumor immunity, including interaction and mobilization of innate immune system representatives. Different antigen-presenting cells migrate to draining lymph nodes and induce T-cell activation mediated by TSAs, generating T-lymphocyte clones with antitumor specificity that will perform their antitumor effects mainly at the tumor site. This process is called the tumor immune cycle (Chen and Mellman 2013). The role of CD4+ is controversial as these cells are defined as "double-edged swords" due to their opposing effects in cancer (Das et al. 2018). Naïve CD4+ T-cells undergo differentiation to

Table 1 Cytotoxic T cells in the pathogenesis of HNSCC

Density (TIL score)	Distribution compartment	Survival improvement	Decrease in recurrence rate	HPV infection status	Study type	References
High	Peripheral	Yes	Yes	N/A	139 cases OSCC	Shimizu et al. (2019)
High	N/A	Yes	N/A	Positive	83 cases TSCC	Näsman et al. (2012)
High	Tumor/stroma	Yes	Yes	Positive	270 cases OPSCC	Ward et al. (2014)
High	Stromal	Yes	Yes	Positive	218 patients OPSCC	Oguejiofor et al. (2017)
High	All	Yes[a]	N/A	Positive	203 cases HNSCC	Ngamphaiboon et al. (2019)

TIL Tumor-infiltrating lymphocyte score, *HPV* Human papillomavirus, *TSCC* Tonsillar squamous cell carcinoma, *OSCC* Oral squamous cell carcinoma, *OPSCC* Oropharyngeal squamous cell carcinoma, *HNSCC* Head and neck squamous cell carcinoma
[a]Concerns non-OPSCC only

activated T helper 1 populations (Th1) in an environment rich in IL-12 or T helper 2 cells (Th2) in the case of a high IL-4 concentration and the absence of IL-12 (Knutson and Disis 2005). Th1 are major antitumor effectors due to cytokine secretion and activation of tumor cell receptors that initiate cell death. Th1 cells act via IFN-γ and TNF-α to induce cancer cells into senescence and initiate their apoptosis (Braumüller et al. 2013). They regulate cytotoxic immune responses and contribute to tumor suppression. Increased expression of specific Th1 cell genetic markers in TME correlates with a good prognosis (Bindea et al. 2013). Some studies suggest that CD4+ T-cells can eliminate tumor cells, in the absence of CD8+ T-cell-mediated immunity, but the cooperation of both cell lines increases the efficiency of antitumor immunity (Fukunaga et al. 2004). In the case of HNSCC, data are not conclusive and often inconsistent regarding CD4+ T-cells. A study assessing the infiltration of CD8+ and CD4+ T-cells in HNSCC has failed to find any relationship of CD4+ T-cells with survival or the HPV status (Nordfors et al. 2013). Different results have been reported in another study where patients exhibiting a high density of activated CD4+ T-cells had better survival and improved local control (Badoual et al. 2006). A meta-analysis assessing prognostic correlations of different types of TILs in HNSCC has reported favorable outcomes in tumors with high TILs for both CD3+ and CD8+ T-cells but failed to find significant correlations for CD4+ T-cells (de Ruiter et al. 2017). The difficulty in assessing prognostic properties of CD4+ T-cells probably has to do with the subgroups of cells that have antagonistic effects in cancer. Regulatory T-cells (Treg Foxp3+) have been intensively studied and are suspected to promote tumorigenesis through immunosuppressive effects. In normal conditions, Tregs, marked with CD25+ and transcription factor Foxp3+, are responsible for maintaining immune tolerance and autoimmunity prevention (Sakaguchi 2005). Increased expression of Treg markers in TME and peripheral circulation is often associated with tumor progression. Tregs show inhibitory effects on CD4+, CD8+, and dendritic cells, inducing immune cell exhaustion through cytokine release, like TGF-β or IL-10 (Bauer et al. 2014; Jarnicki et al. 2006).

In some cancers, TME displays an immunosuppressive effect on CD4+ T-cells by stimulating their differentiation into the Treg subtype (Zheng et al. 2009). In cutaneous SCC, disease aggressiveness correlates with a high density of Treg cells and increased concentrations of IL-10 and TGF-β (Azzimonti et al. 2015). However, contrasting results have been reported for HNSCC where tumor infiltration with FoxP3+

T-cells is identified in patients with improved prognosis (de Ruiter et al. 2017). A similar favorable prognostic correlation for intense Treg infiltration has been reported in colorectal cancers (Salama et al. 2009). The innate immune system has been widely studied in cancers, along with adaptive immunity.

Natural Killer (NK) Cells These cells are the main representatives of innate immunity and are considered equivalents of cytotoxic T-cells in the adaptive immune system. NK cells trigger death in infected or cancer cells via the release of enzymes, perforins, and cytokines, like TNF family members (Spits et al. 2016). Tumor cells have protection mechanisms against innate immunity that rely on TGF-β release with alterations in cytotoxic abilities of NK cells (Cortez et al. 2017). Immature NK cells (CD3-CD56brightCD16-) are activated by cytokines and IFN-γ. Mature NK cells (CD3-CD56dimCD16+) release cytoplasmic inclusions with enzymes and perforins that act directly on malignant cells inducing their lysis. CD16+ receptor expressed on NK cells binds with tumor cells through IgG molecules initiating their activation. Co-activatory stimuli, such as IL-2, IL-12, IL-15, IL-18, and IFN-γ are necessary to induce NK cell cytotoxic function leading to malignant cell clearance (Hu et al. 2019; Minetto et al. 2019). These molecules can be detected in TME. High concentrations of activated NK cells as a complementary defense system, alongside immunity mediated by T and B lymphocytes, has been associated with better outcomes (Nair and Dhodapkar 2017). Tumor cells use protective mechanisms against being recognized by NK cells. Denaturation of peptide constituents from specific ligands affects NK receptor interaction, altering the NK-mediated immune defense (de Andrade et al. 2018).

Lymphocytes B There is a debate regarding the role of lymphocyte B infiltrates in cancers. Studies in experimental models have shown that in genetically modified mice with depletion of lymphocytes B, there is no progression to epithelial malignancies (de Visser et al. 2005). In HNSCC, a correlation has been reported between the HPV status and B cell population, with prognostic potential. Patients with an intense lymphocyte B infiltrate alongside CD8+ cells have a significantly improved prognosis. It is suggested that activated B cells release the chemokine (C-X-C motif) ligand 9 (CXCL9) cytokine that supports the recruitment of CD8+ lymphocytes, promoting tumor cell clearance (Hladíková et al. 2019). The role of B cells in HNSCC pathogenesis has been emphasized in another study that reports high intra-tumoral percentages of antigen-presenting, activated, and memory B cells (Lechner et al. 2019). These findings encourage further research and support the potential role of B cells as new therapeutic targets in HNSCC.

Tumor-Associated Macrophages (TAM) High densities of tumor-associated macrophages (TAMs) were identified in many cancers, including epithelial malignancies, acting as tumor-promoting agents (Li et al. 2020). TAMs release VEGF and MMP, facilitating angiogenesis, local invasion, and metastasis (Evrard et al. 2019). In advanced HNSCC, in patients with enhanced immune profile with associating high densities of TAM, signaling for immune checkpoint ligands is upregulated, which also correlates with poor prognosis (Cao et al. 2017). A recent meta-analysis has reported that a high density of TAMs in HNSCC is associated with advanced tumors, nodal staging, and vascular and lymphatic invasion (Kumar et al. 2019). Refinement of TAM detection, which seems of prognostic significance, is suggested in another meta-analysis. Immunosuppressive subtype M2 of TAMs (CD163+) strongly correlates with a worse prognosis in patients with HNSCC (Troiano et al. 2019).

Antigen-Presenting Cells (APC) These cells play an important role in carcinogenesis. TSAs are presented through the MHC, initiating an adaptive immune response with the generation of antigen-specific T-cell clones (Bottomley et al. 2019). In HNSCC, dendritic cells (DCs) act as APCs together with lymphocytes B, TAMs, and other immune cells (Wondergem et al. 2020). There are contradictory data concerning DCs and their influence on the prognosis in HNSCC, with some studies reporting a favorable outcome in association with a high density of DCs (Jardim et al. 2018) while others report opposing results (Hilly et al. 2016).

4.4 Immune Checkpoints in HNSCC

The complexity and diversity of TME and the multitude of interactions between all its elements make it hard for the scientific community to unveil many of its mysteries. A recent discovery of immune checkpoint molecules has revolutionized the world of immunology and pathophysiology in cancer and enriched the pallet of cancer therapies with an innovative approach through immune checkpoint inhibitors.

In advanced HNSCC, an enhanced immune cell infiltrate often exhibited overexpression of checkpoint molecules. These molecules, which normally act as a protection mechanism against excessive immune reactions and autoimmunity, have a negative influence on cancers. Signaling pathways initiated through the checkpoint molecules weaken the reactivity of T-cells and induce an anergic status known as "immune exhaustion". It can affect both CD4+ and CD8+ T-cells and is reversible under the action of checkpoint blockade therapies, rendering back function to exhausted immune cells (Ostroumov et al. 2018).

Cytotoxic T lymphocyte antigen 4 (CTLA-4), expressed mainly by T-cells, is a transmembrane protein with affinity for B7 molecules, expressed on APCs. B7 molecules, represented by two subtypes CD80 and CD86, bind with CD28 expressed on T-cells, with costimulatory action in addition to TCR activation (Carreno and Collins 2002). The binding of CD80/CD86 to the costimulatory receptor CD28 activates T lymphocytes with simultaneous overexpression of CTLA4 (Mei et al. 2020). Competitive binding of CTLA4 to B7 molecules, due to a higher affinity of CTLA4 for CD80/CD86 rather than for CD28, induces T-cell exhaustion and an overall effect of immunosuppression (Postow et al. 2015).

Programmed cell death protein-1 (PD-1), expressed on activated immune cells, has a negative regulatory effect on T-cells, after binding to its specific ligands, PD-L1 and PD-L2, present on tumor and immune cells (Mei et al. 2020). This leads to an intracellular signaling blockade that interferes with normal activation and proliferation of T-cells (Alsaab et al. 2017). However, studies have shown that in different malignancies, through repeated mutations, clones of immune cells resistant to PD-1 blockade are selected (Hugo et al. 2016; Koyama et al. 2016). Expression of PD-1 and PD-L1 in HNSCC is influenced by the inflammatory cytokines IFN-γ and TNF-α and shows high dynamics, which can explain resistance to immunotherapy (Oguejiofor et al. 2017). PD-1 and PD-L1 are also considered the key players in the initiation and progression of HPV-induced HNSCC (Lyford-Pike et al. 2013). The prognostic value of PD-L1 has been suggested in a study on 203 patients with HNSCC showing a high infiltration with CD8+ in correlation with improved overall survival. However, patients with moderate and high expression of PD-L1 have a worse prognosis compared to those with low PD-L1 expression, defined as less than 1% (Ngamphaiboon et al. 2019).

Immune exhaustion affecting CD4+ T-cells features an overexpression of inhibiting coreceptors, like T-cell immunoglobulin mucin-3 (TIM-3). The binding of TIM-3 with the specific ligand galactin-9 induces CD4+ T-cell apoptosis and a functional deficit in CD8+ T-cells (Mei et al. 2020). Studies in experimental models have reported an increased tumor recurrence rate associated with immune exhaustion of CD4+ T-cells, suggesting that combined immune therapies would be more effective in controlling recurrent malignancies (Koyama et al. 2016). Exhausted immune cells are characterized by alteration of proliferation, cytokine secretion, and deficient recognition of specific antigens. The clinical expression of immune exhaustion is tumor progression and recurrence (Xia et al.

2019). The heterogenic character of HNSCC raises challenges in immunotherapy research due mainly to etiological and immunological differences that require an individualized approach for each patient (Perri et al. 2020).

5 Biomarkers in the Management of HNSCC

The determination of immune biomarkers may significantly influence the management of cancer patients. The prognostic feature of biomarkers in cancers could allow the stratification of patients into risk groups, facilitating early identification of patients with resistance to therapy or aggressive disease. Also, the potential of repeated measurements when analyzing circulating biomarkers assists the patient monitoring and provides early notification of tumor progression. Unraveling the mechanisms of antitumor immunity is one of the steps in the identification of new therapeutic targets that may guide and modulate the antitumor immune response.

In HNSCC, as in many cancers, biomarkers are an emerging subject of interest. Studies have revealed a large number of molecules that promise to predict prognosis, resistance to therapy, or recurrence (Tampa et al. 2018b). Our research group has extensively studied neuroendocrine factors as potential HNSCC biomarkers that can further clarify the pathogenesis and disease progression (Solomon et al. 2018; Lupu et al. 2017). Currently, prognosis in HNSCC is mainly dictated by clinical staging and primary location. Therefore, 5-year survival rates can be higher than 90% in the early stages of lower lip tumors and drop below 40% in advanced oral tumors with distant metastasis (Hladíková et al. 2019). The tumor HPV status is another marker with confirmed prognostic potential in many studies (Kobayashi et al. 2018, Chakravarthy et al. 2016), although one study identified a subset of HPV-positive tumors that did not differ in terms of prognosis from HPV-negative disease (Ward et al. 2014). Local and systemic antitumor immunity has been intensively assessed as biomarkers in HNSCC. Tumor-infiltrating lymphocytes (TILs) have been identified as prognostic markers independent of HPV status, and an increased density of TILs and CD8+ T-cells correlates with higher survival rates (Heikkinen et al. 2019; de Ruiter et al. 2017; Distel et al. 2009). A quick semiquantitative method for evaluating TILs, called TILws (weight sum score), facilitates their use as prognostic biomarkers in the clinical setting (Spector et al. 2019).

6 Emerging Therapies for HNSCC Patients

The increased interest for antitumor immunity has sparked, following the observation that the stimulation of immune elements caused tumor regression even in advanced disease stages. Therefore, immune system modulation has been intensively investigated and became a part of the anticancer arsenal, with outstanding results in some types of neoplasia (Dobosz and Dzieciątkowski 2019; Trapani and Darcy 2017).

Standard treatment in HNSCC consists of surgery, radiotherapy, or a combination of the two and is guided by disease staging and anatomical location, disregarding biological characteristics of the tumor. Early stages (I and II) may be treated by surgical resection or radiotherapy, with similar results in disease control. Combined therapy is recommended in advanced stage II and stage III cases. Standard therapy includes resection of cervical lymph nodes or extended neck radiotherapy (National Cancer Institute 2015). Neoadjuvant chemotherapy is investigated in locally advanced diseases and the TPF regimen (docetaxel, cisplatin, and fluorouracil) improves local disease control and prognosis after surgery (Haddad et al. 2018). A 4% increase in the survival rate has been reported when chemo- and radiotherapy are combined in unresectable advanced disease (Pignon et al. 2001).

Immunotherapy and target therapy for advanced and metastatic HNSCC have been recently approved. These therapies mediate the activation or reactivation of the immune system by modulating its antitumor effects. The first targeted therapy approved by the Food and Drug

Administration (FDA) and the European Medicines Agency for the treatment of recurrent and metastatic disease was cetuximab, an inhibitor of epidermal growth factor receptors (EGFR). Cetuximab added to chemotherapy increases the response rate to treatment by 13% in HNSCC (Vermorken et al. 2008). In 2019, the same regulatory institutions approved the use of anti-PD1 monoclonal antibodies, nivolumab and pembrolizumab, for treatment of recurrent and metastatic disease in chemoresistant patients. These agents block PD-1 receptors overexpressed on T-cells and prevent specific ligand binding, such as PD-L1 and PD-L2 expressed by tumor cells, which exert inhibitory effects on immune cells (Xia et al. 2019). Pembrolizumab is approved as the first-line therapy in association with chemotherapy in patients with metastatic or unresectable disease but can also be administered alone in tumors with PD-L1 overexpression, with a combined positive score of ≥ 1 (Cohen et al. 2019a). Other therapeutic regimens of monoclonal antibodies are under review for advanced HNSCC. For instance, a human monoclonal antibody against CTLA-4, tremelimumab, prevents binding of the inhibiting receptor CTLA4 expressed on immune cells with the specific ligands CD86 and CD80. CTLA4 blockers act on Treg cells inducing their depletion and increasing the ratio of effector-to-Treg cells (Selby et al. 2013). Phase III study EAGLE has evaluated the association between a new anti-PD1 agent, durvalumab, and tremelimumab in patients with metastatic and recurrent disease, reporting no significant differences in survival rates compared to the group receiving cetuximab and chemotherapy (Ferris et al. 2020). Molecules that stimulate NK-mediated immunity are also studied in patients with HNSCC as they are the main effectors in antitumor defense, alongside CD8+ T-cells. Monalizumab is the first member of this class that acts on the natural killer cell receptor (NKG2A) expressed by CD8+ and NK cells present in TME. Preliminary results from an ongoing study investigating the association of monalizumab and cetuximab in 40 patients with recurrent or metastatic disease are encouraging (Cohen et al. 2019b). NK-activating interleukins are also studied as potential therapeutic agents in HNSCC. Infusion of IL-2 in experimental models led to severe adverse reactions and an exponential increase of Tregs inducing antitumor tolerance, invalidating any potential benefits in repelling cancer (Nelson 2004). Infusion of NK cells has been experimentally attempted, and when associated with IL-15 it determined complete tumor regression (Miller et al. 2005). Treg expansion induced by IL-2 might be overcome through the administration of IL-15. Preclinical studies have shown that IL-15 can activate NK and CD8+ T-cells without inducing Treg expansion (Waldmann 2015). Studies evaluating the effects of IL-15 administration have reported a significant increase in NK cells and, secondary, in CD8 + T-cells that additionally contribute to increasing NK cell density through a CD16-mediated pathway (Miller and Lanier 2019; Nair and Dhodapkar 2017).

HNSCC prevention is also of major interest, especially considering the increased incidence of HPV-related disease. As global anti-smoking campaigns induced a decrease in smoking-related HNSCC (Rettig and D'Souza 2015), anti-HPV vaccination is anticipated to yield similar results. A series of vaccines targeting HPV-positive HNSCCs is under testing, and preliminary results support their role in preventing the progression of dysplasia to cancer (Wang et al. 2018). Intratumor injection of viral agents is also investigated in advanced HNSCC (Old et al. 2016), after good results in the treatment of malignant melanoma have been reported, which led to FDA approval of oncolytic virus, talimogene, in this malignancy (Bommareddy et al. 2017). HNSCC is accessible for this type of therapy, and the reported effects on circulating T-cells in patients with solid tumors that do not respond to treatment support the role of viral therapy in fighting cancer by stimulating the antitumor immune response (Taipale et al. 2015). Thus, there are outstanding prospects for preventing and curing oncological ailments. HNSCC is regarded with a great interest for emerging therapies that will advance the management of this disease.

7 Conclusions

Major improvements in disease control and survival in HNSCC have been correlated with staging. Thus, early diagnosis is of paramount importance to detect patients at high risk of an unfavorable outcome, allowing the appropriate therapeutic approach. Numerous studies have shown that inflammation is a key player in HNSCC progression, regardless of cancer location and the main risk factors involved. Moreover, immunity has been highlighted as a major factor in disease control. Further studies in this area of research will allow unveiling new mechanisms in the complex connections between immuno-inflammatory processes and carcinogenesis and will open new possibilities to identify more reliable and widely applicable predictive factors and therapeutic targets in HNSCC.

Acknowledgments Funded by the following grants from the Romanian Ministry of Education and Research Program CCCDI-UEFISCDI: PCCDI/2018 PN-III-P1-1.2-PCCDI-2017-0341 (project number 61) and PN-III-P1-1.2-PCCDI-2017-0062 (contract no. 58)/component project no. 2, within PNCDI-III; Program 1 - The Improvement of the National System of Research and Development, Subprogram 1.2 - Institutional Excellence - Projects of Excellence Funding in RDI, Contract No. 7PFE/16.10.2018; Core Program PN 19.29.01.04.

Conflicts of Interest The authors declare no conflicts of interest concerning this chapter.

Ethical Approval This chapter does not contain any studies with human participants or animals performed by any of the authors.

References

Aggarwal B, Sethi G, Nair A, Ichikawa H (2006) Nuclear factor-κB: a holy grail in cancer prevention and therapy. Curr Signal Transduction Ther 1(1):25–52

Alfred G, Knudson J (1971) Mutation and cancer: statistical study of retinoblastoma. Proc Natl Acad Sci U S A 68:820–823

Allin KH, Bojesen SE, Nordestgaard BG (2009) Baseline C-reactive protein is associated with incident cancer and survival in patients with cancer. J Clin Oncol 27 (13):2217–2224

Alsaab HO, Sau S, Alzhrani R, Tatiparti K, Bhise K, Kashaw SK, Iyer AK (2017) PD-1 and PD-L1 checkpoint signaling inhibition for cancer immunotherapy: mechanism, combinations, and clinical outcome. Front Pharmacol 8:561

Alsibai KD, Meseure D (2018) Significance of tumor microenvironment scoring and immune biomarkers in patient stratification and cancer outcomes. In: Histopathology. IntechOpen, Rijeka. https://doi.org/10.5772/intechopen.72648. Accessed on 14 Jan 2021

Amin MB, Greene FL, Edge SB, Compton CC, Gershenwald JE, Brookland RK, Meyer L, Gress DM, Byrd DR, Winchester DP (2017) The Eighth Edition AJCC Cancer Staging Manual: continuing to build a bridge from a population-based to a more "personalized" approach to cancer staging. CA Cancer J Clin 67(2):93–99

Anderson KG, Stromnes IM, Greenberg PD (2017) Obstacles posed by the tumor microenvironment to T cell activity: a case for synergistic therapies. Cancer Cell 31(3):311–325

Antunes DA, Devaurs D, Moll M, Lizée G, Kavraki LE (2018) General prediction of peptide-MHC binding modes using incremental docking: a proof of concept. Sci Rep 8(1):4327

Asegaonkar SB, Asegaonkar BN, Takalkar UV, Advani S, Thorat AP (2015) C-reactive protein and breast cancer: new insights from old molecule. Int J Breast Cancer 2015:145647

Aziz S, Ahmed SS, Ali A, Khan FA, Zulfiqar G, Iqbal J, Khan AA, Shoaib M (2015) Salivary immunosuppressive cytokines IL-10 and IL-13 are significantly elevated in oral squamous cell carcinoma patients. Cancer Investig 33(7):318–328

Azzimonti B, Zavattaro E, Provasi M, Vidali M, Conca A, Catalano E, Rimondini L, Colombo E, Valente G (2015) Intense Foxp3+ CD25+ regulatory T cell infiltration is associated with high-grade cutaneous squamous cell carcinoma and counterbalanced by CD8+/Foxp3+ CD25+ ratio. Br J Dermatol 172:64–73

Badoual C, Hans S, Rodriguez J, Peyrard S, Klein C, Agueznay Nel H, Mosseri V, Laccourreye O, Bruneval P, Fridman WH, Brasnu DF, Tartour E (2006) Prognostic value of tumor-infiltrating CD4+ T-cell subpopulations in head and neck cancers. Clin Cancer Res 12(2):465–472

Balkwill F, Coussens LM (2004) Cancer: an inflammatory link. Nature 431(7007):405–406

Bauer CA, Kim EY, Marangoni F, Carrizosa E, Claudio NM, Mempel TR (2014) Dynamic Treg interactions with intratumoral APCs promote local CTL dysfunction. J Clin Invest 124(6):2425–2440

Bharti AC, Aggarwal BB (2002) Nuclear factor-kappa B and cancer: its role in prevention and therapy. Biochem Pharmacol 64(5–6):883–888

Bindea G, Mlecnik B, Tosolini M, Kirilovsky A, Waldner M, Obenauf AC, Angell H, Fredriksen T, Lafontaine L, Berger A, Bruneval P, Fridman WH, Becker C, Pagès F, Speicher MR, Trajanoski Z, Galon J (2013) Spatiotemporal dynamics of intratumoral immune cells reveal the immune landscape in human cancer. Immunity 39(4):782–795

Boda D, Neagu M, Constantin C, Voinescu RN, Caruntu C, Zurac S, Spandidos DA, Drakoulis N, Tsoukalas D, Tsatsakis AM (2016) HPV strain distribution in patients with genital warts in a female population sample. Oncol Lett 12(3):1779–1782

Boda D, Docea AO, Calina D, Ilie MA, Caruntu C, Zurac S, Neagu M, Constantin C, Branisteanu DE, Voiculescu V, Mamoulakis C, Tzanakakis G, Spandidos DA, Drakoulis N, Tsatsakis AM (2018) Human papilloma virus: apprehending the link with carcinogenesis and unveiling new research avenues (review). Int J Oncol 52(3):637–655

Bommareddy PK, Patel A, Hossain S, Kaufman HL (2017) Talimogene laherparepvec (T-VEC) and other oncolytic viruses for the treatment of melanoma. Am J Clin Dermatol 18(1):1–15

Bottomley MJ, Thomson J, Harwood C, Leigh I (2019) The role of the immune system in cutaneous squamous cell carcinoma. Int J Mol Sci 20(8):2009

Braumüller H, Wieder T, Brenner E, Aßmann S, Hahn M, Alkhaled M, Schilbach K, Essmann F, Kneilling M, Griessinger C, Ranta F, Ullrich S, Mocikat R, Braungart K, Mehra T, Fehrenbacher B, Berdel J, Niessner H, Meier F, van den Broek M, Häring HU, Handgretinger R, Quintanilla-Martinez L, Fend F, Pesic M, Bauer J, Zender L, Schaller M, Schulze-Osthoff K, Röcken M (2013) T-helper-1-cell cytokines drive cancer into senescence. Nature 494 (7437):361–365

Cai DL, Jin LP (2017) Immune cell population in ovarian tumor microenvironment. J Cancer 8(15):2915–2923

Calcinotto A, Filipazzi P, Grioni M, Iero M, De Milito A, Ricupito A, Cova A, Canese R, Jachetti E, Rossetti M, Huber V, Parmiani G, Generoso L, Santinami M, Borghi M, Fais S, Bellone M, Rivoltini L (2012) Modulation of microenvironment acidity reverses anergy in human and murine tumor-infiltrating T lymphocytes. Cancer Res 72(11):2746–2756

Calenic B, Greabu M, Caruntu C, Tanase C, Battino M (2015) Oral keratinocyte stem/progenitor cells: specific markers, molecular signaling pathways and potential uses. Periodontol 69(1):68–82

Campo-Trapero J, Cano-Sánchez J, Palacios-Sánchez B, Llamas-Martínez S, Lo Muzio L, Bascones-Martínez A (2008) Cellular senescence in oral cancer and precancer and treatment implications: a review. Acta Oncol 47(8):1464–1474

Cancer Genome Atlas Network (2015) Comprehensive genomic characterization of head and neck squamous cell carcinomas. Nature 517(7536):576–582

Cao B, Wang Q, Zhang H, Zhu G, Lang J (2017) Two immune-enhanced molecular subtypes differ in inflammation, checkpoint signaling and outcome of advanced head and neck squamous cell carcinoma. Onco Targets Ther 7(2):e1392427

Carreno BM, Collins M (2002) The B7 family of ligands and its receptors: new pathways for costimulation and inhibition of immune responses. Annu Rev Immunol 20:29–53

Castellanos MR, Pan Q (2016) Novel p53 therapies for head and neck cancer. World J Otorhinolaryngol Head Neck Surg 2:68–75

Chakravarthy A, Henderson S, Thirdborough SM, Ottensmeier CH, Su X, Lechner M, Feber A, Thomas GJ, Fenton TR (2016) Human papillomavirus drives tumor development throughout the head and neck: improved prognosis is associated with an immune response largely restricted to the oropharynx. J Clin Oncol 34:4132–4141

Chalmers ZR, Connelly CF, Fabrizio D et al (2017) Analysis of 100,000 human cancer genomes reveals the landscape of tumor mutational burden. Genome Med 9:1–14

Chan JW, Yeh I, El-Sayed IH, Algazi AP, Glastonbury CM, Ha PK, Yom SS, van Zante A (2019) Ultraviolet light-related DNA damage mutation signature distinguishes cutaneous from mucosal or other origin for head and neck squamous cell carcinoma of unknown primary site. Head Neck 41:E82–E85

Chen DS, Mellman I (2013) Oncology meets immunology: the cancer-immunity cycle. Immunity 39(1):1–10

Chen CJ, Sung WW, Su TC, Chen MK, Wu PR, Yeh KT, Ko JL, Lee H (2013) High expression of interleukin 10 might predict poor prognosis in early stage oral squamous cell carcinoma patients. Clin Chim Acta 415:25–30

Chi AC, Day TA, Neville BW (2015) Oral cavity and oropharyngeal squamous cell carcinoma-an update. CA Cancer J Clin 65:401–421

Cohen EEW, Bell RB, Bifulco CB, Burtness B, Gillison ML, Harrington KJ, Le QT, Lee NY, Leidner R, Lewis RL, Licitra L, Mehanna H, Mell LK, Raben A, Sikora AG, Uppaluri R, Whitworth F, Zandberg DP, Ferris RL (2019a) The Society for Immunotherapy of Cancer consensus statement on immunotherapy for the treatment of squamous cell carcinoma of the head and neck (HNSCC). J Immunother Cancer 7:1–31

Cohen RB, Lefebvre G, Posner MR, Bauman JR, Salas S, Even C, Saada-Bouzid E, Seiwert T, Colevas D, Calmels F, Zerbib R, André P, Boyer-Chammard A, Fayette J (2019b) Monalizumab in combination with cetuximab in patients (pts) with recurrent or metastatic (R/M) head and neck cancer (SCCHN) previously treated or not with PD-(L)1 inhibitors (IO): 1-year survival data. Ann Oncol 30(Suppl_5):v449–v474. https://doi.org/10.1093/annonc/mdz252

Coley WB (1910) The treatment of inoperable sarcoma by bacterial toxins (the mixed toxins of the Streptococcus erysipelas and the Bacillus prodigiosus). Proc R Soc Med 3(Surg Sect):1–48

Cortez VS, Ulland TK, Cervantes-Barragan L, Bando JK, Robinette ML, Wang Q, White AJ, Gilfillan S, Cella M, Colonna M (2017) SMAD4 impedes the conversion of NK cells into ILC1-like cells by curtailing non-canonical TGF-β signaling. Nat Immunol 18(9):995–1003

Cruz-Gregorio A, Aranda-Rivera AK, Aparicio-Trejo OE, Coronado-Martínez I, Pedraza-Chaverri J, Lizano M (2019) E6 oncoproteins from high-risk human papillomavirus induce mitochondrial metabolism in a head and neck squamous cell carcinoma model. Biomol Ther 9(8):351

Das D, Sarkar B, Mukhopadhyay S, Banerjee C, Mondal SB (2018) An altered ratio of CD4+ and CD8+ T lymphocytes in cervical cancer tissues and peripheral blood – a prognostic clue? Asian Pac J Cancer Prev 19:471–478

Dayyani F, Etzel CJ, Liu M, Ho CH, Lippman SM, Tsao AS (2010) Meta-analysis of the impact of human papillomavirus (HPV) on cancer risk and overall survival in head and neck squamous cell carcinomas (HNSCC). Head Neck Oncol 2:1–11

de Andrade LF, En Tay R, Pan D, Luoma AM, Ito Y, Badrinath S, Tsoucas D, Franz B, May KF Jr, Harvey CJ, Kobold S, Pyrdol JW, Yoon C, Yuan GC, Hodi FS, Dranoff G, Wucherpfennig KW (2018) Antibody-mediated inhibition of MICA and MICB shedding promotes NK cell-driven tumor immunity. Science 59 (6383):1537–1542

de Ruiter EJ, Ooft ML, Devriese LA, Willems SM (2017) The prognostic role of tumor infiltrating T-lymphocytes in squamous cell carcinoma of the head and neck: a systematic review and meta-analysis. Onco Targets Ther 6:1–10

de Visser KE, Korets LV, Coussens LM (2005) De novo carcinogenesis promoted by chronic inflammation is B lymphocyte dependent. Cancer Cell 7(5):411–423

Denaro N, Lo Nigro C, Natoli G, Russi EG, Adamo V, Merlano MC (2011) The role of p53 and MDM2 in head and neck cancer. ISRN Otolaryngol 2011:931813

Dinarello CA (2000) Proinflammatory cytokines. Chest 118(2):503–508

Distel LV, Fickenscher R, Dietel K, Hung A, Iro H, Zenk J, Nkenke E, Büttner M, Niedobitek G, Grabenbauer GG (2009) Tumour infiltrating lymphocytes in squamous cell carcinoma of the oro- and hypopharynx: prognostic impact may depend on type of treatment and stage of disease. Oral Oncol 45 (10):e167–e174

Dobosz P, Dzieciątkowski T (2019) The intriguing history of cancer immunotherapy. Front Immunol 10:2965

Doorbar J, Egawa N, Griffin H, Kranjec C, Murakami I (2015) Human papillomavirus molecular biology and disease association. Rev Med Virol 25(Suppl Suppl 1):2–23

Dudley ME, Yang JC, Sherry R, Hughes MS, Royal R, Kammula U, Robbins PF, Huang J, Citrin DE, Leitman SF, Wunderlich J, Restifo NP, Thomasian A, Downey SG, Smith FO, Klapper J, Morton K, Laurencot C, White DE, Rosenberg SA (2008) Adoptive cell therapy for patients with metastatic melanoma: evaluation of intensive myeloablative chemoradiation preparative regimens. J Clin Oncol 26(32):5233–5239

Duesberg PH, Vogt PK (1970) Differences between the ribonucleic acids of transforming and nontransforming avian tumor viruses. Proc Natl Acad Sci U S A 67:1673–1680

Economopoulou P, Psyrri A (2017) Epidemiology, risk factors and pathogenesis of squamous cell tumours. In Head and Neck Cancers: Essentials for clinicians. https://oncologypro.esmo.org/content/download/113133/1971849/file/2017-ESMO-Essentials-for-Clinicians-Head-Neck-Cancers-Chapter-1.pdf

Elgart K, Faden DL (2020) Sinonasal squamous cell carcinoma: etiology, pathogenesis, and the role of human papilloma virus. Curr Otorhinolaryngol Rep 8:111–119

Evrard D, Szturz P, Tijeras-Raballand A, Astorgues-Xerri-L, Abitbol C, Paradis V, Raymond E, Albert S, Barry B, Faivre S (2019) Macrophages in the microenvironment of head and neck cancer: potential targets for cancer therapy. Oral Oncol 88:29–38

Fancello L, Gandini S, Pelicci PG, Mazzarella L (2019) Tumor mutational burden quantification from targeted gene panels: major advancements and challenges. J Immunother Cancer 7(1):183

Faraji F, Zaidi M, Fakhry C, Gaykalova DA (2017) Molecular mechanisms of human papillomavirus-related carcinogenesis in head and neck cancer. Microbes Infect 19:464–475

Farhan-Alanie OM, McMahon J, McMillan DC (2015) Systemic inflammatory response and survival in patients undergoing curative resection of oral squamous cell carcinoma. Br J Oral Maxillofac Surg 53 (2):126–131

Feller L, Chandran R, Khammissa RAG, Meyerov R, Lemmer J (2013) Alcohol and oral squamous cell carcinoma. SADJ 68:176–180

Ferris RL, Haddad R, Even C, Tahara M, Dvorkin M, Ciuleanu TE, Clement PM, Mesia R, Kutukova S, Zholudeva L, Daste A, Caballero-Daroqui J, Keam B, Vynnychenko I, Lafond C, Shetty J, Mann H, Fan J, Wildsmith S, Morsli N, Fayette J, Licitra L (2020) Durvalumab with or without tremelimumab in patients with recurrent or metastatic head and neck squamous cell carcinoma: EAGLE, a randomized, open-label phase III study. Ann Oncol 31(7):942–950

Fukunaga A, Miyamoto M, Cho Y, Murakami S, Kawarada Y, Oshikiri T, Kato K, Kurokawa T, Suzuoki M, Nakakubo Y, Hiraoka K, Itoh T, Morikawa T, Okushiba S, Kondo S, Katoh H (2004) CD8+ tumor-infiltrating lymphocytes together with CD4+ tumor-infiltrating lymphocytes and dendritic cells improve the prognosis of patients with pancreatic adenocarcinoma. Pancreas 28(1):e26–e31

Gameiro SF, Ghasemi F, Barrett JW, Koropatnick J, Nichols AC, Mymryk JS, Maleki Vareki S (2018)

Treatment-naïve HPV+ head and neck cancers display a T-cell-inflamed phenotype distinct from their HPV- counterparts that has implications for immunotherapy. Onco Targets Ther 7(10):e1498439
Gameiro SF, Ghasemi F, Barrett JW, Nichols AC, Mymryk JS (2019) High level expression of MHC-II in HPV+ head and neck cancers suggests that tumor epithelial cells serve an important role as accessory antigen presenting cells. Cancers (Basel) 11(8):1129
Garrido F (2019) MHC/HLA class I loss in cancer cells. Adv Exp Med Biol 1151:15–78
Georgescu SR, Sârbu MI, Matei C, Ilie MA, Caruntu C, Constantin C, Neagu M, Tampa M (2017) Capsaicin: friend or foe in skin cancer and other related malignancies? Nutrients 9(12):1365
Georgescu SR, Mitran CI, Mitran MI, Caruntu C, Sarbu MI, Matei C, Nicolae I, Tocut SM, Popa MI, Tampa M (2018) New insights in the pathogenesis of HPV infection and the associated carcinogenic processes: the role of chronic inflammation and oxidative stress. J Immunol Res 2018:5315816
Georgescu SR, Tampa M, Mitran CI, Mitran MI, Caruntu C, Caruntu A, Lupu M, Matei C, Constantin C, Neagu M (2020) Tumor microenvironment in skin carcinogenesis. Adv Exp Med Biol 1226:123–142
Grafetstätter M, Hüsing A, González Maldonado S, Sookthai D, Johnson T, Pletsch-Borba L, Katzke VA, Hoffmeister M, Bugert P, Kaaks R, Kühn T (2019) Plasma fibrinogen and sP-selectin are associated with the risk of lung cancer in a prospective study. Cancer Epidemiol Biomark Prev 28(7):1221–1227
Greten FR, Grivennikov SI (2019) Inflammation and cancer: triggers, mechanisms, and consequences. Immunity 51:27–41
Haddad RI, Posner M, Hitt R, Cohen EEW, Schulten J, Lefebvre JL, Vermorken JB (2018) Induction chemotherapy in locally advanced squamous cell carcinoma of the head and neck: role, controversy, and future directions. Ann Oncol 29:1130–1140
Hanahan D, Weinberg RA (2011) Hallmarks of cancer: the next generation. Cell 144:646–674
Hanai N, Sawabe M, Kimura T, Suzuki H, Ozawa T, Hirakawa H, Fukuda Y, Hasegawa Y (2018) The high-sensitivity modified Glasgow prognostic score is superior to the modified Glasgow prognostic score as a prognostic predictor for head and neck cancer. Oncotarget 9:37008–37016
Hashibe M, Brennan P, Benhamou S et al (2007) Alcohol drinking in never users of tobacco, cigarette smoking in never drinkers, and the risk of head and neck cancer: pooled analysis in the international head and neck cancer epidemiology consortium. J Natl Cancer Inst 99(10):777–789
Heikkinen I, Bello IO, Wahab A et al (2019) Assessment of tumor-infiltrating lymphocytes predicts the behavior of early-stage oral tongue cancer. Am J Surg Pathol 43:1392–1396
Hilly O, Strenov Y, Rath-Wolfson L, Hod R, Shkedy Y, Mizrachi A, Koren R, Shpitzer T (2016) The predictive value of dendritic cells in early squamous cell carcinoma of the tongue. Pathol Res Pract 212 (12):1138–1143
Hladíková K, Koucký V, Bouček J, Laco J, Grega M, Hodek M, Zábrodský M, Vošmik M, Rozkošová K, Vošmiková H, Čelakovský P, Chrobok V, Ryška A, Špíšek R, Fialová A (2019) Tumor-infiltrating B cells affect the progression of oropharyngeal squamous cell carcinoma via cell-to-cell interactions with CD8+ T-cells. J Immunother Cancer 7(1):1–16
Holzinger D, Danilovic I, Seemann R, Kornek G, Engelmann J, Pillerstorff R, Holawe S, Psyrri A, Erovic BM, Farwell G, Perisanidis C (2016) Prognostic impact of pretreatment plasma fibrinogen in patients with locally advanced oral and oropharyngeal cancer. PLoS One 11(6):e0158697
Hosseini M, Kasraian Z, Rezvani HR (2017) Energy metabolism in skin cancers: a therapeutic perspective. Biochim Biophys Acta Bioenerg 1858:712–722
Hu W, Wang G, Huang D, Sui M, Xu Y (2019) Cancer immunotherapy based on natural killer cells: current progress and new opportunities. Front Immunol 10:1–16
Hugo W, Zaretsky JM, Sun L, Song C, Moreno BH, Hu-Lieskovan S, Berent-Maoz B, Pang J, Chmielowski B, Cherry G, Seja E, Lomeli S, Kong X, Kelley MC, Sosman JA, Johnson DB, Ribas A, Lo RS (2016) Genomic and transcriptomic features of response to anti-PD-1 therapy in metastatic melanoma. Cell 165(1):35–44
Husain N, Neyaz A (2017) Human papillomavirus associated head and neck squamous cell carcinoma: controversies and new concepts. J Oral Biol Craniofac Res 7(3):198–205
Ibrahim-Hashim A, Estrella V (2019) Acidosis and cancer: from mechanism to neutralization. Cancer Metastasis Rev 38:149–155
International Human Genome Sequencing Consortium (2004) Finishing the euchromatic sequence of the human genome. Nature 431(7011):931–945
Jardim JF, Gondak R, Galvis MM, Pinto CAL, Kowalski LP (2018) A decreased peritumoral CD1a+ cell number predicts a worse prognosis in oral squamous cell carcinoma. Histopathology 72(6):905–913
Jarnicki AG, Lysaght J, Todryk S, Mills KHG (2006) Suppression of antitumor immunity by IL-10 and TGF-β-producing T cells infiltrating the growing tumor: influence of tumor environment on the induction of CD4+ and CD8+ regulatory T cells. J Immunol 177(2):896–904
Jiang X, Wu J, Wang J, Huang R (2019) Tobacco and oral squamous cell carcinoma: a review of carcinogenic pathways. Tob Induc Dis 17:29
Jinno T, Kawano S, Maruse Y, Matsubara R, Goto Y, Sakamoto T, Hashiguchi Y, Kaneko N, Tanaka H, Kitamura R, Toyoshima T, Jinno A, Moriyama M, Oobu K, Kiyoshima T, Nakamura S (2015) Increased

expression of interleukin-6 predicts poor response to chemoradiotherapy and unfavorable prognosis in oral squamous cell carcinoma. Oncol Rep 33 (5):2161–2168

Johnson SD, Levingston C, Young MRI (2016) Premalignant oral lesion cells elicit increased cytokine production and activation of T-cells. Anticancer Res 36 (7):3261–3270

Jou A, Hess J (2017) Epidemiology and molecular biology of head and neck Cancer. Oncol Res Treat 40:328–332

Karpathiou G, Vieville M, Gavid M, Camy F, Dumollard JM, Magné N, Froudarakis M, Prades JM, Peoc'h M (2019) Prognostic significance of tumor budding, tumor-stroma ratio, cell nests size, and stroma type in laryngeal and pharyngeal squamous cell carcinomas. Head Neck 41:1918–1927

Kärre K (2008) Natural killer cell recognition of missing self. Nat Immunol 9(5):477–480

Keck MK, Zuo Z, Khattri A, Stricker TP, Brown CD, Imanguli M, Rieke D, Endhardt K, Fang P, Brägelmann J, DeBoer R, El-Dinali M, Aktolga S, Lei Z, Tan P, Rozen SG, Salgia R, Weichselbaum RR, Lingen MW, Story MD, Ang KK, Cohen EE, White KP, Vokes EE, Seiwert TY (2015) Integrative analysis of head and neck cancer identifies two biologically distinct HPV and three non-HPV subtypes. Clin Cancer Res 21(4):870–881

Kersten K, de Visser KE, van Miltenburg MH, Jonkers J (2017) Genetically engineered mouse models in oncology research and cancer medicine. EMBO Mol Med 9 (2):137–153

Khandavilli SD, Ceallaigh PÓ, Lloyd CJ, Whitaker R (2009) Serum C-reactive protein as a prognostic indicator in patients with oral squamous cell carcinoma. Oral Oncol 45(10):912–914

Khowal S, Wajid S (2019) Role of smoking-mediated molecular events in the genesis of oral cancers. Toxicol Mech Methods 29(9):665–685

Kim SM (2016) Human papilloma virus in oral cancer. J Korean Assoc Oral Maxillofac Surg 42:327

Knutson KL, Disis ML (2005) Augmenting T helper cell immunity in cancer. Curr Drug Targets Immune Endocr Metabol Disord 5:365–371

Kobayashi K, Hisamatsu K, Suzui N, Hara A, Tomita H, Miyazaki T (2018) A review of HPV-related head and neck cancer. J Clin Med 7(9):241

Koebel CM, Vermi W, Swann JB, Zerafa N, Rodig SJ, Old LJ, Smyth MJ, Schreiber RD (2007) Adaptive immunity maintains occult cancer in an equilibrium state. Nature 450(7171):903–907

Koyama S, Akbay EA, Li YY, Taube JM, Westra WH, Akpeng B, Bruno TC, Richmon JD, Wang H, Bishop JA, Chen L, Drake CG, Topalian SL, Pardoll DM, Pai SI (2016) Adaptive resistance to therapeutic PD-1 blockade is associated with upregulation of alternative immune checkpoints. Nat Commun 7:1–9

Kuilman T, Michaloglou C, Vredeveld LCW, Douma S, van Doorn R, Desmet CJ, Aarden LA, Mooi WJ, Peeper DS (2008) Oncogene-induced senescence relayed by an interleukin-dependent inflammatory network. Cell 133:1019–1031

Kuilman T, Michaloglou C, Mooi WJ, Peeper DS (2010) The essence of senescence. Genes Dev 24:2463–2479

Kumar AT, Knops A, Swendseid B, Martinez-Outschoom U, Harshyne L, Philp N, Rodeck U, Luginbuhl A, Cognetti D, Johnson J, Curry J (2019) Prognostic significance of tumor-associated macrophage content in head and neck squamous cell carcinoma: a meta-analysis. Front Oncol 9:656

Lan M, Chen C, Huang Y, Mao M, Han F, Liao J, Deng M, Duan Z, Zheng L, Wu S, Lu T, Jian Y (2016) Elevated plasma fibrinogen level shows superior prognostic value than Epstein-Barr virus DNA load for stage IVA/B nasopharyngeal carcinoma patients in the intensity-modulated radiotherapy era. Oncotarget 7 (29):46242–46252

Lechner A, Schlößer HA, Thelen M, Wennhold K, Rothschild SI, Gilles R, Quaas A, Siefer OG, Huebbers CU, Cukuroglu E, Göke J, Hillmer A, Gathof B, Meyer MF, Klussmann JP, Shimabukuro-Vornhagen A, Theurich S, Beutner D, von Bergwelt-Baildon M (2019) Tumor-associated B cells and humoral immune response in head and neck squamous cell carcinoma. Onco Targets Ther 8:1535293

Li J, Wang J, Chen R, Bai Y, Lu X (2017) The prognostic value of tumor-infiltrating T lymphocytes in ovarian cancer. Oncotarget 8:15621–15631

Li B, Ren M, Zhou X, Han Q, Cheng L (2020) Targeting tumor-associated macrophages in head and neck squamous cell carcinoma. Oral Oncol 106:104723

Lupu M, Caruntu A, Caruntu C, Papagheorghe LML, Ilie MA, Voiculescu V, Boda D, Constantin C, Tanase C, Sifaki M, Drakoulis N, Mamoulakis C, Tzanakakis G, Neagu M, Spandidos DA, Izotov BN, Tsatsakis AM (2017) Neuroendocrine factors: the missing link in non-melanoma skin cancer (review). Oncol Rep 38 (3):1327–1340

Lupu M, Caruntu A, Caruntu C, Boda D, Moraru L, Voiculescu V, Bastian A (2018a) Non-invasive imaging of actinic cheilitis and squamous cell carcinoma of the lip. Mol Clin Oncol 8(5):640–646

Lupu M, Căruntu ANA, Moraru L, Voiculescu VM, Boda D, Tănase C, Căruntu C (2018b) Non-invasive imaging techniques for early diagnosis of radiation-induced squamous cell carcinoma of the lip. Romanian J Morphol Embryol 59:949–953

Lupu M, Caruntu A, Boda D, Caruntu C (2020) *In vivo* reflectance confocal microscopy-diagnostic criteria for actinic cheilitis and squamous cell carcinoma of the lip. J Clin Med 9(6):1987

Lyford-Pike S, Peng S, Young GD et al (2013) Evidence for a role of the PD-1:PD-L1 pathway in immune resistance of HPV-associated head and neck squamous cell carcinoma. Cancer Res 73(6):1733–1741

Lyu H, Li M, Jiang Z, Liu Z, Wang X (2019) Correlate the TP53 mutation and the HRAS mutation with immune signatures in head and neck squamous cell cancer. Comput Struct Biotechnol J 17:1020–1030

Markowska J, Markowska A (1998) Spontaneous tumor regression. Ginekol Pol 69:39–44

Mazzaschi G, Madeddu D, Falco A, Bocchialini G, Goldoni M, Sogni F, Armani G, Lagrasta CA, Lorusso B, Mangiaracina C, Vilella R, Frati C, Alfieri R, Ampollini L, Veneziani M, Silini EM, Ardizzoni A, Urbanek K, Aversa F, Quaini F, Tiseo M (2018) Low PD-1 expression in cytotoxic CD8+ tumor-Infiltrating lymphocytes confers an immune-privileged tissue microenvironment in NSCLC with a prognostic and predictive value. Clin Cancer Res 24 (2):407–419

McGranahan N, Furness AJS, Rosenthal R et al (2016) Clonal neoantigens elicit T cell immunoreactivity and sensitivity to immune checkpoint blockade. Science 351(6280):1463–1469

McManus JF (1958) Rudolf Virchow in 1858. Lab Investig 7:549–553

Mei Z, Huang J, Qiao B, Lam AK (2020) Immune checkpoint pathways in immunotherapy for head and neck squamous cell carcinoma. Int J Oral Sci 12(1):16

Miller JS, Lanier LL (2019) Natural killer cells in cancer immunotherapy. Annu Rev Cancer Biol 3:77–103

Miller JS, Soignier Y, Panoskaltsis-Mortari A, McNearney SA, Yun GH, Fautsch SK, McKenna D, Le C, Defor TE, Burns LJ, Orchard PJ, Blazar BR, Wagner JE, Slungaard A, Weisdorf DJ, Okazaki IJ, McGlave PB (2005) Successful adoptive transfer and *in vivo* expansion of human haploidentical NK cells in patients with cancer. Blood 105(8):3051–3057

Minetto P, Guolo F, Pesce S, Greppi M, Obino V, Ferretti E, Sivori S, Genova C, Lemoli RM, Marcenaro E (2019) Harnessing NK cells for cancer treatment. Front Immunol 10:2836

Mittal D, Gubin MM, Schreiber RD, Smyth MJ (2014) New insights into cancer immunoediting and its three component phases-elimination, equilibrium and escape. Curr Opin Immunol 27:16–25

Monisha J, Roy NK, Bordoloi D, Kumar A, Golla R, Kotoky J, Padmavathi G, Kunnumakkara AB (2017) Nuclear factor kappa B: a potential target to persecute head and neck cancer. Curr Drug Targets 18:232–253

Morgan RA, Dudley ME, Wunderlich JR, Hughes MS, Yang JC, Sherry RM, Royal RE, Topalian SL, Kammula US, Restifo NP, Zheng Z, Nahvi A, de Vries CR, Rogers-Freezer LJ, Mavroukakis SA, Rosenberg SA (2006) Cancer regression in patients after transfer of gentically engineered lymphocytes. Science 314(5796):126–129

Mosesson MW (2005) Fibrinogen and fibrin structure and functions. J Thromb Haemost 3(8):1894–1904

Nair S, Dhodapkar MV (2017) Natural killer T-cells in cancer immunotherapy. Front Immunol 8:1–27

Näsman A, Romanitan M, Nordfors C, Grün N, Johansson H, Hammarstedt L, Marklund L, Munck-Wikland E, Dalianis T, Ramqvist T (2012) Tumor infiltrating CD8+ and Foxp3+ lymphocytes correlate to clinical outcome and human papillomavirus (HPV) status in tonsillar cancer. PLoS One 7:1–8

National Cancer Institute (2015) Head and neck cancer. Lip and oral cavity cancer treatment (adult) (PDQ®) – Health Professional Version. https://www.cancer.gov/types/head-and-neck/hp/adult/lip-mouth-treatment-pdq. Accessed on 12 Jan 2021

Ndiaye C, Mena M, Alemany L, Arbyn M, Castellsagué X, Laporte L, Bosch FX, de Sanjosé S, Trottier H (2014) HPV DNA, E6/E7 mRNA, and p16INK4a detection in head and neck cancers: a systematic review and meta-analysis. Lancet Oncol 15:1319–1331

Neagu M, Caruntu C, Constantin C, Boda D, Zurac S, Spandidos DA, Tsatsakis AM (2016) Chemically induced skin carcinogenesis: updates in experimental models (review). Oncol Rep 35(5):2516–2528

Neagu M, Constantin C, Caruntu C, Dumitru C, Surcel M, Zurac S (2019) Inflammation: a key process in skin tumorigenesis (review). Oncol Lett 17(5):4068–4084

Nelson BH (2004) IL-2, regulatory T cells, and tolerance. J Immunol 172(7):3983–3988

Ngamphaiboon N, Chureemas T, Siripoon T, Arsa L, Trachu N, Jiarpinitnun C, Pattaranutaporn P, Sirachainan E, Larbcharoensub N (2019) Characteristics and impact of programmed death-ligand 1 expression, CD8+ tumor-infiltrating lymphocytes, and p16 status in head and neck squamous cell carcinoma. Med Oncol 36:21

NIH (2017) National Institutes of Health – National Cancer Institute. Cancer Stat Facts: Oral Cavity and Pharynx Cancer. https://seer.cancer.gov/statfacts/html/oralcav.html. Accessed on 10 Jan 2021

Nordfors C, Grün N, Tertipis N, Ährlund-Richter A, Haeggblom L, Sivars L, Du J, Nyberg T, Marklund L, Munck-Wikland E, Näsman A, Ramqvist T, Dalianis T (2013) CD8+ and CD4+ tumour infiltrating lymphocytes in relation to human papillomavirus status and clinical outcome in tonsillar and base of tongue squamous cell carcinoma. Eur J Cancer 49(11):2522–2530

Oguejiofor K, Hall J, Slater C, Betts G, Hall G, Slevin N, Dovedi S, Stern PL, West CML (2015) Stromal infiltration of CD8 T-cells is associated with improved clinical outcome in HPV-positive oropharyngeal squamous carcinoma. Br J Cancer 113(6):886–893

Oguejiofor K, Galletta-Williams H, Dovedi SJ, Roberts DL, Stern PL, West CML (2017) Distinct patterns of infiltrating CD8+ T-cells in HPV+ and CD68 macrophages in HPV- oropharyngeal squamous cell carcinomas are associated with better clinical outcome but PD-L1 expression is not prognostic. Oncotarget 8:14416–14427

Old MO, Wise-Draper T, Wright CL, Kaur B, Teknos T (2016) The current status of oncolytic viral therapy for head and neck cancer. World J Otorhinolaryngol Neck Surg 2(2):84–89

Opitz JM (2016) Annals of morphology THEODOR BOVERI (1862–1915) to commemorate the centenary of his death and contributions to the Sutton–Boveri hypothesis. Am J Med Genet A 170:2803–2829

Ostroumov D, Fekete-Drimusz N, Saborowski M, Kühnel F, Woller N (2018) CD4 and CD8 T lymphocyte interplay in controlling tumor growth. Cell Mol Life Sci 75:689–713

Otsuka M, Egawa G, Kabashima K (2018) Uncovering the mysteries of Langerhans cells, inflammatory dendritic epidermal cells, and monocyte-derived Langerhans cell-like cells in the epidermis. Front Immunol 9:1768

Pan QX, Su ZJ, Zhang JH, Wang CR, Ke SY (2017) Glasgow Prognostic Score predicts prognosis of intrahepatic cholangiocarcinoma. Mol Clin Oncol 6 (4):566–574

Perdrix A, Najem A, Saussez S, Awada A, Journe F, Ghanem G, Krayem M (2017) PRIMA-1 and PRIMA-1Met (APR-246): from mutant/wild type p53 reactivation to unexpected mechanisms underlying their potent anti-tumor effect in combinatorial therapies. Cancers (Basel) 9:1–17

Pérez Sayáns M, Chamorro Petronacci CM, Lorenzo Pouso AI, Padín Iruegas E, Blanco Carrión A, Suárez Peñaranda JM, García García A (2019) Comprehensive genomic review of TCGA head and neck squamous cell carcinomas (HNSCC). J Clin Med 8:1896

Perri F, Pisconti S, Della VSG (2016) P53 mutations and cancer: a tight linkage. Ann Transl Med 4:2–5

Perri F, Ionna F, Longo F, Della Vittoria Scarpati G, De Angelis C, Ottaiano A, Botti G, Caponigro F (2020) Immune response against head and neck cancer: biological mechanisms and implication on therapy. Transl Oncol 13:262–274

Peter F, Wittekindt C, Finkensieper M, Kiehntopf M, Guntinas-Lichius O (2013) Prognostic impact of pretherapeutic laboratory values in head and neck cancer patients. J Cancer Res Clin Oncol 139(1):171–178

Pettersen JS, Fuentes-Duculan J, Suárez-Fariñas M, Pierson KC, Pitts-Kiefer A, Fan L, Belkin DA, Wang CQ, Bhuvanendran S, Johnson-Huang LM, Bluth MJ, Krueger JG, Lowes MA, Carucci JA (2011) Tumor-associated macrophages in the cutaneous SCC microenvironment are heterogeneously activated. J Invest Dermatol 131(6):1322–1330

Pignon J, Bourhis J, Domenge C, Designe L (2001) Chemotherapy added to locoregional treatment for head and neck squamous-cell carcinoma: three meta-analyses of updated individual data. MACH-NC Collaborative Group. Meta-analysis of chemotherapy on head and neck cancer. Lancet 355(9208):949–955

Pilon-Thomas S, Kodumudi KN, El-Kenawi AE, Russell S, Weber AM, Luddy K, Damaghi M, Wojtkowiak JW, Mulé JJ, Ibrahim-Hashim A, Gillies RJ (2016) Neutralization of tumor acidity improves antitumor responses to immunotherapy. Cancer Res 76(6):1381–1390

Postow MA, Callahan MK, Wolchok JD (2015) Immune checkpoint blockade in cancer therapy. J Clin Oncol 33:1974–1982

Punyani SR, Sathawane RS (2013) Salivary level of interleukin-8 in oral precancer and oral squamous cell carcinoma. Clin Oral Investig 17(2):517–524

Quabius ES, Haag J, Kühnel A, Henry H, Hoffmann AS, Görögh T, Hedderich J, Evert M, Beule AG, Maune S, Knecht R, Óvári A, Durisin M, Hoppe F, Tribius S, Röcken C, Ambrosch P, Hoffmann M (2015) Geographical and anatomical influences on human papillomavirus prevalence diversity in head and neck squamous cell carcinoma in Germany. Int J Oncol 46:414–422

Quezada SA, Simpson TR, Peggs KS, Merghoub T, Vider J, Fan X, Blasberg R, Yagita H, Muranski P, Antony PA, Restifo NP, Allison JP (2010) Tumor-reactive CD4+ T-cells develop cytotoxic activity and eradicate large established melanoma after transfer into lymphopenic hosts. J Exp Med 207(3):637–650

Rao SK, Pavicevic Z, Du Z, Kim JG, Fan M, Jiao Y, Rosebush M, Samant S, Gu W, Pfeffer LM, Nosrat CA (2010) Pro-inflammatory genes as biomarkers and therapeutic targets in oral squamous cell carcinoma. J Biol Chem 285(42):32512–32521

Rettig EM, D'Souza G (2015) Epidemiology of head and neck cancer. Surg Oncol Clin N Am 24(3):379–396

Ribatti D (2017) The concept of immune surveillance against tumors. The first theories. Oncotarget 8 (4):7175–7180

Roh JL, Jang H, Kim EH, Shin D (2017) Targeting of the glutathione, thioredoxin, and Nrf2 antioxidant systems in head and neck cancer. Antioxidants Redox Signal 27 (2):106–114

Rooney MS, Shukla SA, Wu CJ, Getz G, Hacohen N (2015) Molecular and genetic properties of tumors associated with local immune cytolytic activity. Cell 160:48–61

Saijo M, Nakamura K, Masuyama H, Ida N, Haruma T, Kusumoto T, Seki N, Hiramatsu Y (2017) Glasgow Prognostic Score is a prognosis predictor for patients with endometrial cancer. Eur J Obstet Gynecol Reprod Biol 210:355–359

Sakaguchi S (2005) Naturally arising Foxp3-expressing CD25+ CD4+ regulatory T-cells in immunological tolerance to self and non-self. Nat Immunol 6 (4):345–352

Salama P, Phillips M, Grieu F, Morris M, Zeps N, Joseph D, Platell C, Iacopetta B (2009) Tumor-infiltrating FOXP3+ T regulatory cells show strong prognostic significance in colorectal cancer. J Clin Oncol 27(2):186–192

Sato J, Ohuchi M, Abe K, Satoh T, Abe T, Yamazaki Y, Satoh A, Notani KI, Kitagawa Y (2013) Correlation between salivary interleukin-6 levels and early locoregional recurrence in patients with oral squamous cell carcinoma: preliminary study. Head Neck 35 (6):889–894

Scheau C, Badarau IA, Mihai LG, Scheau AE, Costache DO, Constantin C, Calina D, Caruntu C, Costache RS, Caruntu A (2020) Cannabinoids in the pathophysiology of skin inflammation. Molecules 25(3):6522

Schiegnitz E, Kämmerer PW, Schön H, Blatt S, Berres M, Sagheb K, Al-Nawas B (2018) Proinflammatory cytokines as serum biomarker in oral carcinoma - a

prospective multi-biomarker approach. J Oral Pathol Med 38:42–49
Schumacher TN, Scheper W, Kvistborg P (2019) Cancer neoantigens. Annu Rev Immunol 37:173–200
Seifi S, Feizi F, Mehdizadeh M, Khafri S, Ahmadi B (2014) Evaluation of cytological alterations of oral mucosa in smokers and waterpipe users. Cell J 15 (4):302–309
Selby MJ, Engelhardt JJ, Quigley M, Henning KA, Chen T, Srinivasan M, Korman AJ (2013) Anti-CTLA-4 antibodies of IgG2a isotype enhance antitumor activity through reduction of intratumoral regulatory T-cells. Cancer Immunol Res 1(1):32–42
Selzer E, Grah A, Heiduschka G, Kornek G, Thurnher D (2016) Pre-therapeutic fibrinogen levels are of prognostic significance in locally advanced head and neck cancer. Wien Klin Wochenschr 128(9–10):320–328
Shimizu S, Hiratsuka H, Koike K, Tsuchihashi K, Sonoda T, Ogi K, Miyakawa A, Kobayashi J, Kaneko T, Igarashi T, Hasegawa T, Miyazaki A (2019) Tumor-infiltrating CD8+ T-cell density is an independent prognostic marker for oral squamous cell carcinoma. Cancer Med 8(1):80–93
Simpson-Haidaris PJ, Rybarczyk B (2001) Tumors and fibrinogen. The role of fibrinogen as an extracellular matrix protein. Ann N Y Acad Sci 936:406–425
Smyth MJ, Dunn GP, Schreiber RD (2006) Cancer immunosurveillance and immunoediting: the roles of immunity in suppressing tumor development and shaping tumor immunogenicity. Adv Immunol 90:1–50
Solomon I, Voiculescu VM, Caruntu C, Lupu M, Popa A, Ilie MA, Albulescu R, Caruntu A, Tanase C, Constantin C, Neagu M, Boda D (2018) Neuroendocrine factors and head and neck squamous cell carcinoma: an affair to remember. Dis Markers 2018:9787831
Spector ME, Bellile E, Amlani L, Zarins K, Smith J, Brenner JC, Rozek L, Nguyen A, Thomas D, McHugh JB, Taylor JMG, Wolf GT (2019) Prognostic value of tumor-infiltrating lymphocytes in head and neck squamous cell carcinoma. JAMA Otolaryngol Head Neck Surg 145(11):1012–1019
Spits H, Bernink JH, Lanier L (2016) NK cells and type 1 innate lymphoid cells: partners in host defense. Nat Immunol 17(7):758–764
Suwanpradid J, Holcomb ZE, MacLeod AS (2017) Emerging skin T-cell functions in response to environmental insults. J Invest Dermatol 137(2):288–294
Tafreshi NK, Lloyd MC, Bui MM, Gillies RJ, Morse DL (2014) Carbonic anhydrase IX as an imaging and therapeutic target for tumors and metastases. Subcell Biochem 75:221–254
Tai SF, Chien HT, Young CK, Tsao CK, de Pablo A, Fan KH, Liao CT, Wang HM, Kang CJ, Chang JT, Huang SF (2017) Roles of preoperative C-reactive protein are more relevant in buccal cancer than other subsites. World J Surg Oncol 15(1):47
Taipale K, Liikanen I, Juhila J, Karioja-Kallio A, Oksanen M, Turkki R, Linder N, Lundin J, Ristimäki A, Kanerva A, Koski A, Joensuu T, Vähä-Koskela M, Hemminki A (2015) T-cell subsets in peripheral blood and tumors of patients treated with oncolytic adenoviruses. Mol Ther 23(5):964–973
Tampa M, Caruntu C, Mitran M, Mitran C, Sarbu I, Rusu LC, Matei C, Constantin C, Neagu M, Georgescu SR (2018a) Markers of oral lichen planus malignant transformation. Dis Markers 2018:1959506
Tampa M, Mitran MI, Mitran CI, Sarbu MI, Matei C, Nicolae I, Caruntu A, Tocut SM, Popa MI, Caruntu C, Georgescu SR (2018b) Mediators of inflammation – a potential source of biomarkers in oral squamous cell carcinoma. J Immunol Res 2018:1061780
Tampa M, Mitran CI, Mitran MI, Nicolae I, Dumitru A, Matei C, Manolescu L, Popa GL, Caruntu C, Georgescu SR (2020) The ROLE OF BEta HPV types and HPV-associated inflammatory processes in cutaneous squamous cell carcinoma. J Immunol Res 2020:5701639
Taniguchi K, Karin M (2018) NF-κB, inflammation, immunity and cancer: coming of age. Nat Rev Immunol 18(5):309–324
Tezal M (2012) Interaction between chronic inflammation and oral HPV infection in the etiology of head and neck cancers. Int J Otolaryngol 2012:575242
Tezal M, Scannapieco FA, Wactawski-Wende J, Hyland A, Marshall JR, Rigual NR, Stoler DL (2012) Local inflammation and human papillomavirus status of head and neck cancers. Arch Otolaryngol Head Neck Surg 138(7):669–675
Thorsson V, Gibbs DL, Brown SD et al (2018) The immune landscape of cancer. Immunity 48 (4):812–830.e14
Trapani JA, Darcy PK (2017) Immunotherapy of cancer. Aust Fam Physician 46(4):194–199
Troiano G, Caponio VCA, Adipietro I, Tepedino M, Santoro R, Laino L, Lo Russo L, Cirillo N, Lo Muzio L (2019) Prognostic significance of CD68+ and CD163+ tumor associated macrophages in head and neck squamous cell carcinoma: a systematic review and meta-analysis. Oral Oncol 93:66–75
Vajdic CM, van Leeuwen MT (2009) Cancer incidence and risk factors after solid organ transplantation. Int J Cancer 125(8):1747–1754
van Pelt GW, Kjær-Frifeldt S, van Krieken JHJM, Al Dieri R, Morreau H, Tollenaar RAEM, Sørensen FB, Mesker WE (2018) Scoring the tumor-stroma ratio in colon cancer: procedure and recommendations. Virchows Arch 473(4):405–412
Vermorken JB, Mesia R, Rivera F, Remenar E, Kawecki A, Rottey S, Erfan J, Zabolotnyy D, Kienzer HR, Cupissol D, Peyrade F, Benasso M, Vynnychenko I, De Raucourt D, Bokemeyer C, Schueler A, Amellal N, Hitt R (2008) Platinum-based chemotherapy plus cetuximab in head and neck cancer. N Engl J Med 359(11):1116–11127
Voiculescu V, Calenic B, Ghita M, Lupu M, Caruntu A, Moraru L, Voiculescu S, Ion A, Greabu M, Ishkitiev N, Caruntu C (2016) From normal skin to squamous cell carcinoma: a quest for novel biomarkers. Dis Markers 2016:4517492

Vomund S, Schäfer A, Parnham MJ, Brüne B, Von Knethen A (2017) Nrf2, the master regulator of anti-oxidative responses. Int J Mol Sci 18:1–19

Waldmann TA (2015) The shared and contrasting roles of IL2 and IL15 in the life and death of normal and neoplastic lymphocytes: implications for cancer therapy. Cancer Immunol Res 3:219–227

Wang YF, Chang SY, Tai SK, Li WY, Wang LS (2002) Clinical significance of interleukin-6 and interleukin-6 receptor expressions in oral squamous cell carcinoma. Head Neck 24(9):850–858

Wang C, Dickie J, Sutavani RV, Pointer C, Thomas GJ, Savelyeva N (2018) Targeting head and neck cancer by vaccination. Front Immunol 9:1–12

Wang J, Sun H, Zeng Q, Guo XJ, Wang H, Liu HH, Dong ZY (2019) HPV-positive status associated with inflamed immune microenvironment and improved response to anti-PD-1 therapy in head and neck squamous cell carcinoma. Sci Rep 9(1):13404

Ward MJ, Thirdborough SM, Mellows T, Riley C, Harris S, Suchak K, Webb A, Hampton C, Patel NN, Randall CJ, Cox HJ, Jogai S, Primrose J, Piper K, Ottensmeier CH, King EV, Thomas GJ (2014) Tumour-infiltrating lymphocytes predict for outcome in HPV-positive oropharyngeal cancer. Br J Cancer 110(2):489–500

Weidhaas JB, Harris J, Schaue D, Chen AM, Chin R, Axelrod R, El-Naggar AK, Singh AK, Galloway TJ, Raben D, Wang D, Matthiesen C, Avizonis VN, Manon RR, Yumen O, Nguyen-Tan PF, Trotti A, Skinner H, Zhang Q, Ferris RL, Sidransky D, Chung CH (2017) The KRAS-variant and cetuximab response in head and neck squamous cell cancer a secondary analysis of a randomized clinical trial. JAMA Oncol 3 (4):483–491

Wellenstein MD, de Visser KE (2018) Cancer-cell-intrinsic mechanisms shaping the tumor immune landscape. Immunity 48:399–416

Wiegand S, Zimmermann A, Wilhelm T, Werner JA (2015) Survival after distant metastasis in head and neck cancer. Anticancer Res 35(10):5499–5502

Wondergem NE, Nauta IH, Muijlwijk T, Leemans CR, van de Ven R (2020) The immune microenvironment in head and neck squamous cell carcinoma: on subsets and subsites. Curr Oncol Rep 22(8):81

Wright TI, Spencer JM, Flowers FP (2006) Chemoprevention of nonmelanoma skin cancer. J Am Acad Dermatol 54(6):933–946

Wu S, Zhu W, Thompson P, Hannun YA (2018) Evaluating intrinsic and non-intrinsic cancer risk factors. Nat Commun 9(1):3490

Xia A, Zhang Y, Xu J, Yin T, Lu XJ (2019) T cell dysfunction in Cancer immunity and immunotherapy. Front Immunol 10:1719

Xu WY, Zhang HH, Yang XB, Bai Y, Lin JZ, Long JY, Xiong JP, Zhang JW, Sang XT, Zhao HT (2018) Prognostic significance of combined preoperative fibrinogen and CA199 in gallbladder cancer patients. World J Gastroenterol 24:1451–1463

Yan M, Xu Q, Zhang P, Zhou XJ, Zhang ZY, Chen WT (2010) Correlation of NF-κB signal pathway with tumor metastasis of human head and neck squamous cell carcinoma. BMC Cancer 10:437

Yang S, Zhao K, Ding X, Jiang H, Lu H (2019) Prognostic significance of hematological markers for patients with nasopharyngeal carcinoma: a meta-analysis. J Cancer 10(11):2568–2577

Zhang JM, An J (2007) Cytokines, inflammation, and pain. Int Anesthesiol Clin 45(2):27–37

Zhang Y, Cao J, Deng Y, Huang Y, Li R, Lin G, Dong M, Huang Z (2020) Pretreatment plasma fibrinogen level as a prognostic biomarker for patients with lung cancer. Clinics (Sao Paulo) 75:e993

Zheng Y, Chaudhry A, Kas A, DeRoos P, Kim JM, Chu TT, Corcoran L, Treuting P, Klein U, Rudensky AY (2009) Regulatory T-cell suppressor program co-opts transcription factor IRF4 to control TH2 responses. Nature 458(7236):351–356

Adv Exp Med Biol - Clinical and Experimental Biomedicine (2022) 13: 37–44
https://doi.org/10.1007/5584_2021_635

Published online: 23 April 2021

Outcome of Repeat Pulmonary Metastasectomy

Marcus Krüger, Katharina Franzke, Taufiek Konrad Rajab, Fabian Nadler, Moritz Möbius-Winkler, Norman Zinne, Daniel Schulz, Miriam Möller, Wolfgang Schütte, Michael Ermitsch, Bassam Redwan, Olaf Schega, and Christian Biancosino

Abstract

Pulmonary metastasectomy is a well-established contribution to the cure of oligometastatic cancers, but its exact effectiveness is poorly understood. Here we report the outcomes of repeat pulmonary metastasectomy from a multicenter trial. This retrospective study included patients who underwent re-do metastasectomies between January 2010 and December 2014. The exclusion criterion was metastasectomy without curative intent. We reviewed medical files of 621 consecutive patients who underwent initial pulmonary metastasectomy. Of those, 64 patients underwent repeat metastasectomies, and these patients were included in the analysis. All the 64 patients underwent a second metastasectomy, later 35 of them underwent a third metastasectomy, 12 underwent a fourth metastasectomy, and 6 underwent a fifth metastasectomy. The total number of re-do

The original version of this chapter was revised: Chapter title was modified. The correction to this chapter is available at https://doi.org/10.1007/5584_2021_650

M. Krüger (✉), M. Möbius-Winkler, M. Möller, and W. Schütte
Department of Thoracic Surgery, Martha – Maria Hospital Halle, Halle, Germany
e-mail: marcus.krueger@martha-maria.de; moritz.moebius-winkler@student.uni-halle.de; miriam.moeller@martha-maria.de; wolfgang.schuette@martha-maria.de

K. Franzke
Department of Internal Medicine, Niels-Stensen-Kliniken Marienhospital Osnabrück, Osnabrück, Germany
e-mail: katharina.franzke@niels-stensen-kliniken.de

T. K. Rajab
Division of Cardiothoracic Surgery, Medical University of South Carolina, Charleston, SC, USA
e-mail: rajabt@musc.edu

F. Nadler, D. Schulz, M. Ermitsch, and O. Schega
Department of Thoracic Surgery, Johanniter Hospital Treuenbrietzen, Treuenbrietzen, Germany
e-mail: fabian-nadler@t-online.de; daniel.schulz@trb.johanniter-kliniken.de; michael.ermitsch@trb.johanniter-kliniken.de; olaf.schega@trb.johanniter-kliniken.de

N. Zinne
Division of Cardiothoracic, Transplantation and Vascular Surgery, Hannover Medical School, Hannover, Germany
e-mail: zinne.norman@mh-hannover.de

B. Redwan
Department of Thoracic Surgery, Klinik am Park Lünen, Lünen, Germany
e-mail: bassam.redwan@klinikum-westfalen.de

C. Biancosino
Department of Thoracic Surgery, HELIOS University Hospital Wuppertal, Wuppertal, Germany
e-mail: christian.biancosino@helios-gesundheit.de

metastasectomies was 181. The median overall survival among the patients undergoing re-do metastasectomy was 66.0 ± 3.8 months. Three and 5-year survival rates were 82.3% and 63.3%, respectively. The 5-year survival rates were 63.3% after the first, 50.9% after the second, 74.4% after the third, 83.3% after the fourth, and 60.0% after the fifth metastasectomy. We conclude that at the current stage of knowledge, there is an indication for repeat re-do metastasectomy with curative intent.

Keywords

Cancer · Lung metastases · Metastasectomy · Pulmonary metastasectomy · Survival

1 Introduction

Pulmonary metastasectomy represents a key therapy option in the treatment of lung metastases, enhancing the chance of long-term survival for selected patients with oligometastatic cancer. Several studies have investigated the benefits of repeated metastasectomy (Yang et al. 2020; Matsumoto et al. 2019; Menna et al. 2018; Salah et al. 2013; Borasio et al. 2011; Welter et al. 2007). Unfortunately, these studies are marred by small numbers of patients, the inclusion of patients from previous eras, or a short follow-up. Mineo et al. (2015) have demonstrated good results following the first re-do metastasectomy, but a less favorable outcome after the second or third re-do procedure. However, that study included patients from the years 1986 to 2010. In the present work, we report the outcomes of re-do metastasectomy in a large, contemporary, multicenter clinical trial.

2 Methods

We retrospectively reviewed the files of 621 consecutive patients who underwent pulmonary metastasectomy at the Johanniter Hospital Treuenbrietzen and Hannover Medical School between January 2010 and December 2014. The criterion for inclusion into the study was re-do metastasectomy. Exclusion criteria were metastasectomies done without curative intent and a loss of follow-ups after metastasectomy, which consisted of checkups with computer tomography (CT) lung scans every 3 months.

The following information was retrieved from patients' files: age at first metastasectomy, gender, primary tumor, nonsurgical oncologic therapies, number of metastases and the largest diameter of metastases, completeness of metastasectomy, lymph node dissection, lymph node metastases, and postoperative complications. Additional follow-up data were obtained from the referring oncologist. A calculation of overall survival (OS) included every alive patient at the time of inclusion. A disease-free interval was defined as the time between the resection of the primary tumor and the first lung metastasectomy. Re-metastasectomy was defined as a lung re-do surgery in patients who had undergone prior pulmonary metastasectomy on the ipsilateral side. In bilateral approaches or bilateral relapse, the side of the first surgery was chosen as a reference. The standard surgical procedure in both clinics was laser metastasectomy. Following anterolateral thoracotomy, bimanual palpation was carried out to detect all metastases. For laser resection, a Neodym:Yag laser Limax 120 using the 1318 nm wavelength (KLS Martin GmbH + Co. KG, Freiburg im Breisgau, Germany) was used. Conventional resections included wedge resections, segmentectomies, lobectomies, and pneumonectomies.

To identify differences between categorical variables, Pearson's c^2 test with Fisher's correction was used. Survival curves were created with the Kaplan Meier method, and survival rates were compared with a log-rank test. To evaluate factors influencing overall survival, the Cox proportional hazards model was applied after empirical variable selection. A p-value of <0.05 defined statistically significant differences.

3 Results

Out of the 621 patients who underwent initial pulmonary metastasectomy, 64 patients aged 62.6 ± 12.8 years (F/M – 28/64) underwent repeat metastasectomy and these patients were included in the analysis (Table 1). The median follow-up was 44 (6–88) months. During the follow-up, 21 patients died. All the patients underwent a second metastasectomy (64/64), later 55% underwent a third metastasectomy (35/64), 19% underwent a fourth metastasectomy (12/64), and 9% underwent a fifth metastasectomy (6/64), bringing a total to 181 of re-do metastasectomies.

The primary malignancies of metastases were colorectal carcinoma 19 (29.7%), renal cell carcinoma 15 (23.4%), sarcoma 9 (14.1%), urothelial carcinoma 4 (6.3%), head and neck cancers 4 (6.3%), and others 13 (20.3%). The median duration from diagnosis of primary malignancy to the first diagnosis of pulmonary metastases was 39.3 (0.0–178.4) months. Of these, 12 patients (18.8%) had a disease-free interval of less than 1 year compared to 10 patients (15.6%) with a disease-free interval of 1–2 years and 42 patients (65.6%) with more than 2 years. Baseline tumor data was regarding the different tumor origins analyzed according to the UICC score grades I–IV. Twenty (31.3%) patients received additional radiation therapy, 4 (6.3%) neoadjuvant, and 23 (35.9%) adjuvant chemotherapy. In 7 (10.9%) patients synchronous liver metastases, and other synchronous metastases were detected in another 8 patients (Table 1).

Two patients received presurgery and four patients received postsurgery chemotherapy for the metastases. Twenty-seven (42.0%) patients developed recurrent metastases after metastasectomy. The sites of metastases were liver (3.1%), brain (3.1%), bone (3.1%), and other localizations (14.1%). Forty-one (64.1%) patients developed pulmonary recurrence after the second surgery, and 35 (54.7%) patients had surgery for the third time. Out of the latter group, 17 (48.6%) patients developed a third pulmonary recurrence and 12 of them (34.3%) underwent a fourth operation. Out of these 12 patients, 6 developed a further recurrence and 3 underwent a fifth operation, with no more recurrences.

The mean number of metastatic nodules resected was 3.3 ± 3.6 and that of histologically confirmed metastases was 2.5 ± 3.0. A solitary metastasis was resected in 74 (40.9%) cases and more than 3 metastases in 46 (25.4%) cases. The median size of metastases was 10.6 ± 24.4 mm. Eighty-six resections were performed on the right side. Staged bilateral approaches were necessary in 79 cases. A complete lymph node dissection was performed in 50% of cases. Five percent of the 970 resected lymph nodes showed malignancy. Postoperative complications occurred in 21 (11.6%) cases. They were prolonged parenchymal fistula lasting for more than 4 days ($n = 12$), pneumothorax ($n = 2$), pneumonia ($n = 2$), respiratory distress ($n = 2$), and other rare complications like pleural effusion, chylothorax, and hemothorax ($n = 3$). The median duration of hospitalization was 9 (3–63) days.

The disease-free intervals were as follows: 19.8 ± 12.6 months after the first lung metastasectomy, 18.6 ± 16.4 months after the second metastasectomy, 19.3 ± 18.7 months after the third metastasectomy, 15.3 ± 14.1 months after the fourth metastasectomy, and 13.5 ± 13.6 months after the fifth metastasectomy.

The univariate Cox-regression analysis determined bilateral metastases, age, gender, resection margin, the number of metastases (>2), synchronous metastases, chemotherapy of the primary tumor, and preoperative liver metastases as significant factors concerning survival. The multivariate analysis determined that the number of metastases of more than two is a negative prognostic factor ($p = 0.013$). This was confirmed in

Table 1 Baseline characteristics of patients with repeat pulmonary metastasectomies

	n (%)
Total	64 (100)
Age (years)	Mean 62.6 ± 12.8
<50	7 (10.9)
50–65	23 (35.9)
>65	34 (53.1)
Gender	
Female	28 (43.8)
Male	36 (56.3)
Disease-free interval	Mean 54.6 ± 49.7
<1 year	12 (18.8)
1–2 years	10 (15.6)
>2 years	42 (65.6)
UICC stage (primary cancer)	41 (64.1)
I	6 (9.4)
II	8 (12.5)
III	16 (25.0)
IV	11 (17.2)
Additional therapy for primary cancer	
Radiotherapy	20 (31.3)
Neoadjuvant chemotherapy	4 (6.3)
Adjuvant chemotherapy	23 (35.9)
Synchronous liver metastases	7 (10.9)

UICC Union for International Cancer Control – cancer staging classification

the Kaplan-Meier curve showing a significantly better survival in the case of fewer than two metastases ($p = 0.0001$) (Fig. 1). The Cox-regression analysis also identified the presence of more than two metastases as a prognostic factor concerning the risk of recurrent lung metastases.

The median overall survival was 66.0 ± 3.8 months, the 1-year survival rate was 100%, the 3-year survival rate was 82.3%, and the 5-year survival rate was 63.3%. The median survival related to the number of resections was 62.2 months after two surgeries, 66.1 months after three surgeries, 73.8 after four surgeries, and 55.8 after five surgeries.

The 5-year overall survival rates were 63.3% after the first surgery, 50.9% after the second surgery, 74.4% after the third surgery, 83.3% after the fourth surgery, and 60.0% after the fifth surgery (Fig. 2). There were no significant differences in survival after the respective number of resections ($p = 0.647$, log-rank test).

4 Discussion

Lung metastasectomy represents a widely accepted therapy option for selected patients with lung metastases originating from a wide range of primary tumors. The concept of oligometastatic recurrence has been invoked to explain good results of local therapeutic approaches despite a metastasized tumor stage (Niibe and Hayakawa 2010; Hellman and Weichselbaum 1995). Like in most other works (Sponholz et al. 2017; Hachimaru et al. 2016; Mizuguchi et al. 2016), in this study, we show that multiple metastasectomies are worthy of performing regarding favorable long-term survival (Table 2). This is consistent with the concept of oligometastasis. If the biology of cancer does not change from the first metastasectomy, then subsequent metastasectomies should have similar efficacy. However, Yang et al. (2020) have described a significantly higher recurrence-

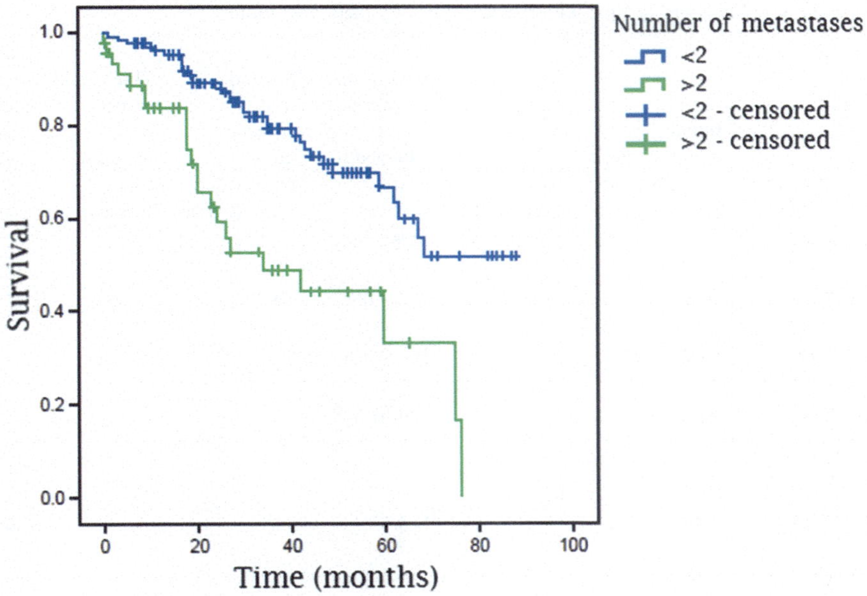

Fig. 1 Survival dependent on the number of metastases (≤2 vs. >2)

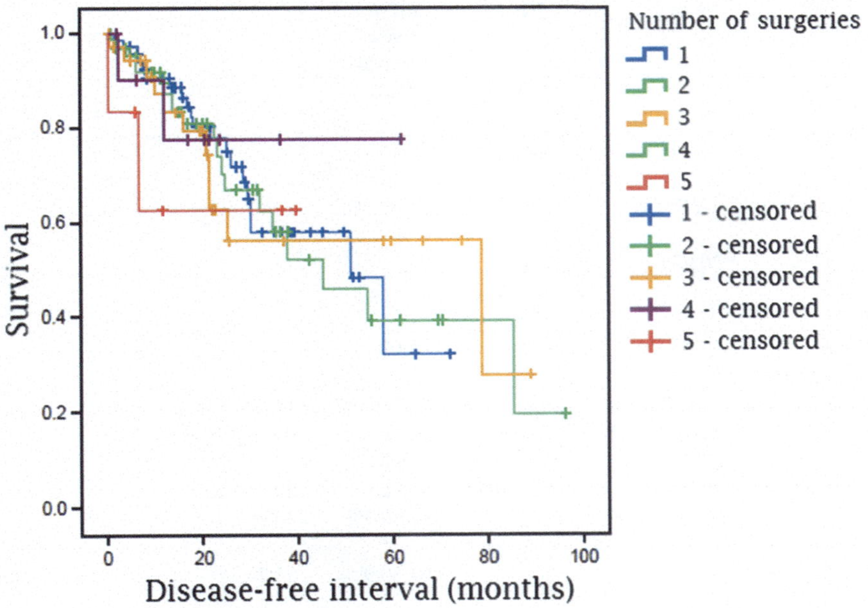

Fig. 2 Five-year overall survival rates depending on the number of metastasectomies

rate following the second re-metastasectomy as 13 out of the 14 patients died or had further recurrences within 12 months following the second re-metastasectomy. The authors conclude that the second metastasectomy is recommended as an optimal therapeutic option for the second recurrence, while further re-metastasectomies should be performed with caution as they may not enhance the survival time. Likewise, Mineo et al. (2015) have performed from two

Table 2 Selection of publications dealing with repeat pulmonary metastasectomies

Authors (year)	Primary tumor	Initial metastasectomy no. of patients/ 5-year survival	First recurrence	First re-do surgery no. of patients/5-year survival	Second re-do surgery no. of patients/5-year survival	Third re-do surgery no. of patients/5-year survival	Fourth re-do surgery no. of patients/5-year survival
Welter et al. (2007)	CRC		169/---	33/53.8%			
Park et al. (2010)	CRC	202/---		48/79.0%	10/78%		
Borasio et al. (2011)	CRC	137/55.4%		16/59.5%	5/---		
Salah et al. (2013) Meta-analysis	CRC	759/58%		148/57.9%			
Mineo et al. (2015)	Various	---/42%		113/65%	54/---	31/---	8/---
Hachimaru et al. (2016)	CRC	138/61.7%		33/64.3%			
Hishida et al. (2017) Multicenter[a]	CRC	898/---	216/898	132/75.3%	22/55.1%	2/---	
Mizuguchi et al. (2016)	HCC	19/48%	7/19	5/67% (3-year survival)			
Chudgar et al. (2017)	STS	539/---	341/539	141/---			
Sponholz et al. (2017)	CRC	238/48%	101/238	52/75%			
Cheung et al. (2018)	Sarcoma	42/20%[b]		20/37.4%[b]	12/63.6%		
Menna et al. (2018) Multicenter	CRC	203/34%		92/[c]	11/---		
Yamamoto et al. (2019)	STS/ osteosarc	44/43.5%		8/60%			
Yang et al. 2020[d]	CRC	248 [d]/74.8% (lung $n = 117$)	133 [d]/248 (lung $n = 58$)	52 [d]/62.8% (lung $n = 31$)	14 [d]/45.6% (lung $n = 9$)		
Matsumoto et al. (2019)[e]	CRC	1073/45% [f] (lung $n = 44$)	809/1073	323 all sites/43%	80 all sites/ 46%		
Present multicenter study	Various	621		64/50.9%	35/74.4%	12/83.3%	6/60.0%

CRC colorectal cancer, *HCC* hepatocellular carcinoma, *STS* soft tissue sarcoma
[a]Nationwide Japanese database
[b]5-year overall survival refers to the patient groups without further metastasectomy
[c]5-year overall survival following repeat metastasectomies showing no significant difference compared to patients with single metastasectomy
[d]Data referring to concomitant lung and liver metastases
[e]Data referring to the concomitant liver, lung, and peritoneal metastases
[f]Number of patients having all recurrences sites (liver, lung, or peritoneum) as opposed to the 5-year overall survival referring to patients with lung metastases only

metastasectomies in 113 patients, three in 51 patients, and so forth down to six re-do metastasectomies in three patients for lung metastases. They found that the more the resections, the greater the probability of recurrences and shorter the disease-free time, possibly making the re-do surgery lose its efficacy after the initial procedure.

A favorable effect on the long-term survival of repeat metastasectomies we found in this review is in line with several other studies. Cheung et al. (2018) have reported an increased median survival of 63.5 months after two and more repeat resections of pulmonary metastases in the sarcoma cohort of 243 patients. Park et al. (2010) have reported that out of 48 patients with colorectal cancer who underwent the second metastasectomy due to pulmonary recurrence, the overall 5-year survival was 79%, and in 10 patients who underwent the third metastasectomy it was 78%. According to Matsumoto et al. (2019), there is no difference concerning the overall 5-year survival following the first and second re-do procedures (43% vs. 46%), whereas Hishida et al. (2017) report a significantly enhanced survival following the first re-do surgery when compared with the second one (75.3% vs. 55.1%) (Table 2).

Presumably, patients with the favorable outcome have not overrun a specific biologic condition of the malignant disease. An interesting issue would be to identify this condition or a threshold over which metastasectomies are of no further benefit. The issue is confounded by differences in prognostic criteria following repeat metastasectomy from one publication to another. According to the present data, more than two metastases were associated with a higher risk of relapse. Other publications dealing with repeat metastasectomy confirm that the number of metastases is a strong negative predictor (Mineo et al. 2015; Salah et al. 2013; Borasio et al. 2011; Welter et al. 2007). Other studies have identified nodal status (Menna et al. 2018), the diameter of the largest metastasis (Yamamoto et al. 2019), concomitant liver metastases (Hishida et al. 2017), or disease-free survival (Yang et al. 2020; Mineo et al. 2015; Borasio et al. 2011) as

Table 3 Significant negative predictors for oncologic outcomes after repeat lung metastasectomies

Authors (year)	Negative predictor 1	Negative predictor 2	Positive predictor
Welter et al. (2007)	Number of metastases		
Borasio et al. (2011)	One vs multiple metastases	DFI <24 months	
Salah et al. (2013)	Number of metastases >3	>3 cm	
Mineo et al. (2015)	Multiple metastases	Short DFI	
Hachimaru et al. (2016)	High serum CEA level prior to re-metastasectomy		
Hishida et al. (2017)	Concomitant liver metastasis	Primary location in the rectum	
Chudgar et al. (2017)[a]	Preoperative chemotherapy prior to re-metastasectomy	R1/R2 metastasectomy	
Sponholz et al. (2017)	Low grading of primary tumor		
Menna et al. (2018)	Nodal status		Adjuvant chemotherapy
Yang et al. (2020)	DFI <6 months		
Yamamoto et al. (2019)	>2 cm (largest nodule)	DFI <12 months	
Present multicenter study	Number of metastases >2		

DFI disease-free interval, *CEA* carcinoembryonic antigen, *R1/R2* resection to microscopic residual tumor/macroscopic residual tumor

[a]Patients with soft tissue sarcoma, a negative predictor for the first re-metastasectomy. Incomplete resection is detected as a negative predictor and is not specifically mentioned in almost all publications

negative predictors as well (Table 3). These data as heterogeneous as are conclusions on metastasectomies in general.

In conclusion, this work supports the notion of a survival benefit of repeat lung metastasectomy. A close interdisciplinary co-operation is of paramount importance for the development of a therapy schedule and the implementation and surveillance of the oncologic treatment. A systematic oncologic follow-up aiming at early detection and consequent local therapy of recurrent metastases may improve survival in selected patients.

Conflicts of Interest The authors declare no conflicts of interest concerning this study.

Ethical Approval This chapter based on a retrospective review of medical files does not contain any direct studies with human participants performed by any of the authors. The work was approved by a local Ethics Committee at Hannover Medical School (IRB no. 2879-2015).

References

Borasio P, Gisabella M, Billé A, Righi L, Longo M, Tampellini M, Ardissone F (2011) Role of surgical resection in colorectal lung metastases: analysis of 137 patients. Int J Color Dis 26(2):183–190

Cheung F, Alam N, Wright G (2018) Pulmonary metastasectomy: analysis of survival and prognostic factors in 243 patients. ANZ J Surg 88(12):1316–1321

Chudgar NP, Brennan MF, Tan KS, Munhoz RR, D'Angelo SP, Bains MS, Huang J, Park BJ, Adusumilli PS, Tap WD, Jones DR (2017) Is repeat pulmonary metastasectomy indicated for soft tissue sarcoma? Ann Thorac Surg 104(6):1837–1845

Hachimaru A, Maeda R, Suda T, Takagi Y (2016) Repeat pulmonary resection for recurrent lung metastases from colorectal cancer: an analysis of prognostic factors. Interact Cardiovasc Thorac Surg 22(6):826–830

Hellman S, Weichselbaum RR (1995) Oligometastases. J Clin Oncol 13:8–10

Hishida T, Tsuboi M, Okumura T, Boku N, Ohde Y, Sakao Y, Yoshiya K, Hyodo I, Mori K, Kondo H (2017) Does repeated lung resection provide long-term survival for recurrent pulmonary metastases of colorectal cancer? Results of a retrospective Japanese Multicenter Study. Ann Thorac Surg 103(2):399–405

Matsumoto T, Hasegawa S, Hida K, Kawada K, Sakai Y, Sugihara K (2019) Role of repeat resection in patients with metastatic colorectal cancer: a multicenter retrospective study. Dis Colon Rectum 62(5):561–567

Menna C, Berardi G, Tierno SM, Andreetti C, Maurizi G, Ciccone AM, D'Andrilli A, Cassiano F, Poggi C, Diso D, Venuta F, Rendina EA, Ibrahim M (2018) Do repeated operations for recurrent colorectal lung metastases result in improved survival? Ann Thorac Surg 106(2):421–427

Mineo TC, Ambrogi V, Tacconi F, Mineo D (2015) Multireoperations for lung metastases. Future Oncol 11 (2 Suppl):37–41

Mizuguchi S, Nishiyama N, Izumi N, Tsukioka T, Komatsu H, Iwata T, Tanaka S, Takemura S, Kubo S (2016) Clinical significance of multiple pulmonary metastasectomy for hepatocellular carcinoma. World J Surg 40(2):380–387

Niibe Y, Hayakawa K (2010) Oligometastases and oligo-recurrence: the new era of cancer therapy. Jpn J Clin Oncol 40:107–111

Park JS, Kim HK, Choi YS, Kim K, Shim YM, Jo J, Lee WY, Chun HK, Park YS, Kang WK, Kim J (2010) Outcomes after repeated resection for recurrent pulmonary metastases from colorectal cancer. Ann Oncol 21 (6):1285–1289

Salah S, Watanabe K, Park JS, Addasi A, Park JW, Zabaleta J, Ardissone F, Kim J, Riquet M, Nojiri K, Gisabella M, Kim SY, Tanaka K (2013) Repeated resection of colorectal cancer pulmonary oligometastases: pooled analysis and prognostic assessment. Ann Surg Oncol 20(6):1955–1961

Sponholz S, Schirren M, Baldes N, Oguzhan S, Schirren J (2017) Repeat resection for recurrent pulmonary metastasis of colorectal cancer. Langenbeck's Arch Surg 402(1):77–85

Welter S, Jacobs J, Krbek T, Stamatis G (2007) Long-term survival after repeated resection of pulmonary metastases from colorectal cancer. Ann Thorac Surg 84(1):203–210

Yamamoto Y, Kanzaki R, Kanou T, Ose N, Funaki S, Shintani Y, Minami M, Outani H, Takenaka S, Hamada K, Yoshikawa H, Okumura M (2019) Long-term outcomes and prognostic factors of pulmonary metastasectomy for osteosarcoma and soft tissue sarcoma. Int J Clin Oncol 24(7):863–870

Yang KM, Park IJ, Lee JL, Kim CW, Yoon YS, Lim SB, Yu CS, Kim JC (2020) Benefits of repeated resections for liver and lung metastases from colorectal cancer. Asian J Surg 43(1):102–109

Adv Exp Med Biol - Clinical and Experimental Biomedicine (2022) 13: 45–51
https://doi.org/10.1007/5584_2020_616

Published online: 14 March 2021

Quality of Life of Patients After Laparoscopic Pyeloplasty Due to Ureteropelvic Junction Obstruction: A Long-Term Observation

Wojciech Panek, Dawid Janczak, Marta Panek, Urszula Szydełko, Rafał Chrzan, Mariusz Chabowski, and Tomasz Szydełko

Abstract

This study aims to define the quality of life (QoL) of patients who had undergone laparoscopic pyeloplasty due to ureteropelvic junction obstruction. The QoL was investigated in 26 patients after pyeloplasty, on average, at a 7.5-year follow-up. The operation was performed in a single center between 2002 and 2009 and its effectiveness was confirmed by diuretic renography. The QoL was assessed using the World Health Organization Quality of Life (WHOQOL-BREF) questionnaire. Additionally, we used an own questionnaire, created for this study, specifically assessing the health-related quality of life after pyeloplasty. Overall, 96% of patients were satisfied with the surgical procedure and all would agree to have another pyeloplasty procedure if needed. In one case, dissatisfaction was caused by persisting postoperative pain. All patients but one, dissatisfied due to persisting pain, reported that the postoperative pain intensity was not a problem that would impact the QoL or professional activity. We conclude that laparoscopic pyeloplasty did not adversely affect the patients' QoL, which might stem from beneficial functional outcomes making the patients satisfied with treatment results.

Keywords

Laparoscopy · Pain · Pyeloplasty · Quality of life · Ureteropelvic obstruction

W. Panek, D. Janczak, and T. Szydełko
Department of Urology, Fourth Military Hospital, Wroclaw, Poland

Division of Oncology and Palliative Care, Faculty of Health Science, Wroclaw Medical University, Wroclaw, Poland

M. Panek
Department of Urology, Fourth Military Hospital, Wroclaw, Poland

U. Szydełko
Department and Clinic of Ophthalmology, Wroclaw Medical University, Wroclaw, Poland

R. Chrzan
Department of Pediatric Urology, Collegium Medicum of the Jagiellonian University, Cracow, Poland

M. Chabowski (✉)
Division of Oncology and Palliative Care, Faculty of Health Science, Wroclaw Medical University, Wroclaw, Poland

Department of Surgery, Fourth Military Teaching Hospital, Wroclaw, Poland

1 Introduction

Minimally invasive surgical techniques gradually replace open surgery. Pyeloplasty is an example of progress. The first laparoscopic pyeloplasty was performed in 1993 (Kavoussi and Peters 1993; Schuessler et al. 1993), and since then the procedure has become the gold standard of treatment. Its clinical effectiveness has been confirmed in many a study (Strother and Mucksavage 2016; Autorino et al. 2014; García-Aparicio et al. 2014; Knoedler et al. 2013).

Currently, increasing attention is placed on the assessment of treatment effectiveness concerning the patient quality of life (QoL) in addition to the functional or survival results. There are often instances when the QoL declines despite improvements in laboratory indices or survival. The ureteropelvic junction obstruction is a common cause requiring laparoscopic pyeloplasty, surgical treatment of choice, but data on the postoperative QoL is scarce (Khoder et al. 2014; Parekh et al. 2008; Sahai et al. 2007). Therefore, in this study, we set out to define the health-related QoL in patients treated with laparoscopy for ureteropelvic junction obstruction at a long-term follow-up. We addressed the issue using the World Health Organization Quality of Life (WHOQOL-BREF) questionnaire, an abbreviated generic Quality of Life Scale, a tool that has not yet been used for this specific surgical entity, with the addition of an own health-related quality of life questionnaire, specifically addressing the after-pyeloplasty condition, created for this study.

2 Methods

Ninety-five patients who underwent transperitoneal unilateral laparoscopic pyeloplasty were originally invited to participate in the study. The time from surgery to the study follow-up visit was at least 5 years, with a mean of 89.8 ± 25.5 months. Twenty-seven patients responded to the invitation, but one of them having a horseshoe kidney was excluded from the study. The patient data were retrospectively obtained from hospital records. The elective surgery was performed in a single center by the same surgeon (TS) between 2002 and 2009, according to internationally recognized techniques (Panek et al. 2019; Krajewski et al. 2017; Szydełko et al. 2010, 2012). The Anderson-Hynes pyeloplasty was performed in 19 (73%), Y-V pyeloplasty in 6 (23%), and Fenger pyeloplasty in 1 patient (4%). The decision regarding the pyeloplasty method was made intraoperatively after visualization of the anatomy of the ureteropelvic junction area.

2.1 Description of Surgical Procedures

Twenty-three patients were symptomatic with hydronephrosis. Three patients with ureteropelvic junction obstruction and hydronephrosis were asymptomatic. Before surgery, patients had undergone preoperative examinations such as ultrasonography, diuretic renography, excretory intravenous urography (IVU), and computed tomography (CT) to confirm the diagnosis of ureteropelvic junction obstruction. The upper limit of the half-time tracer clearance was 12 min for nonobstructive and 20 min for obstructive systems in diuretic renography in which the diuretic furosemide (1 mg/kg/dose) was given after radionuclide administration at the times indicated above. The Foley catheter was removed on the second postoperative day. The closed suction drain was removed 1 day later providing that the drainage was <25 ml per day. The double-J stent was removed 4–6 weeks after pyeloplasty.

2.2 Follow-Up Visit Several Years After Pyeloplasty

At the scheduled follow-up visit, we evaluated each patient's medical history, such as the presence of arterial hypertension, metabolic diseases, or renal and diuresis complaints, and collected information on the passed perioperative period, with emphasis on postoperative complications, according to the classification by Dindo et al.

(2004). We asked patients to estimate the intensity of pain before surgery on a visual analog scale (VAS) of pain. The ruler-scale was 100 mm in length, with a score ranging from 0 mm (no pain) to 100 mm (extreme pain). The following cut-off distances were used: no pain (0–4 mm), mild pain (5–44 mm), moderate pain (45–74 mm), and severe pain (75–100 mm) (Hawker et al. 2011). We assessed the current pain intensity and performed an ultrasound examination of the affected kidney. Each patient was asked to fill out two questionnaires. The main questionnaire was the WHOQOL-BREF, version 1996, consisting of 26 questions. Two questions concern the general quality of life and health status. The remaining ones are divided into four domains: somatic, psychological, social, and environmental. All questions refer to the patient's feelings during the past 4 weeks. The numerical score of each domain reflects the perception of the quality of life represented by the domain. Two patients failed to complete the questionnaire. The other questionnaire was created for this study by one of the authors (WP) and consisted of five items specifically assessing the health-related quality of life after pyeloplasty. It consisted of five items:

1. Are you satisfied with the surgery outcome?
2. Would you agree to have another laparoscopic pyeloplasty if needed?
3. How do you estimate your current pain complaints on the VAS?
4. Does pain significantly affect your life and professional activity?
5. How many additional procedures did you undergo in the aftermath of laparoscopic pyeloplasty?

Besides completing the questionnaires, the patients underwent diuretic renography using the protocol akin to that used before pyeloplasty and the following blood tests: complete blood count, electrolytes, creatinine level, and the estimated glomerular filtration rate.

The pain associated with ureteropelvic junction obstruction before laparoscopic pyeloplasty was retrospectively rated and compared to the pain level on the VAS during the current follow-up visit. Continuous data were expressed as means±SD and differences between the mean values were evaluated using a *t*-test. Categorical data were expressed as counts and percentages. A p-value < 0.05 defined a statistically significant difference. The QoL was assessed after the laparoscopic pyeloplasty only.

3 Results

Out of the 26 patients participating in the study, 10 (38.5%) were men and 16 (61.5%) were women. The mean age at the time of surgery was 32.2 ± 10.6 years (range 16–56 years). In 12 (46.2%) patients, the crossing blood vessels were identified. They are aberrant vessels running to the lower pole of the kidney crossing the ipsilateral ureter most often anteriorly, which causes extrinsic compression of the ureter and obstruction of the renal collecting system. The patients' perioperative characteristics are presented in Table 1.

During the 6-week postoperative time, one significant complication of peritonitis was observed which was caused by a urine leak treated by subsequent laparotomy. Additionally, four patients required a change of a double-J stent. Other complications were infrequent and mild as detailed in Table 2.

In 23 out of the 26 study patients, the half-time tracer clearance was less than 12 min in diuretic renography performed during the study follow-up visit. Surgery resulted in a significant decrease in the perception of pain when voiding reported on the VAS, 6.5 ± 3.5 before to 1.4 ± 1.7 points after pyeloplasty ($p = 0.002$). Detailed follow-up outcomes are presented in Table 3.

Overall, 96% of patients were satisfied with the pyeloplasty procedure and would agree to repeat it if needed, despite that some suffered from postoperative complications. In one case, dissatisfaction was caused by an insufficient decrease in pain. All the patients reported that the low-grade pain persisting post-surgery did not significantly affect their life and professional activity. One patient underwent treatment of renal stones on the operated side a year after

Table 1 Perioperative characteristics concerning laparoscopic pyeloplasty

Sex; n (%)	Male	10 (38.5)
	Female	16 (61.5)
Surgery method; n (%)	Anderson-Hynes pyeloplasty	19 (73.0)
	Y-V pyeloplasty	6 (23.0)
	Fenger pyeloplasty	1 (4.0)
Kidney involved; n (%)	Left	14 (53.8)
	Right	12 (46.2)
Crossing vessels; n (%)	Present	12 (46.2)
	Absent	14 (53.8)
Surgery length; mean ± SD (min)	With crossing vessels	185.0 ± 36.1
	Without crossing vessels	203.2 ± 87.4
	Anderson-Hynes pyeloplasty	207.6 ± 70.3
	Y-V pyeloplasty	166.7 ± 51.3
	Fenger pyeloplasty	120.0
	Average duration of pyeloplasty	194.8 ± 68.0

Table 2 Postoperative complications after laparoscopic pyeloplasty in patients with ureteropelvic junction obstruction, according to the Clavien-Dindo classification of severity

Clavien-Dindo-grade	n (%)	Description	Treatment
I	5 (19.2%)	3 patients (11.5%) – pyrexia	Antipyretics
		2 patients (7.7%) – spontaneous prolapse of a double-J catheter	No treatment
II	1 (3.9)	Asymptomatic urinary infection	Antibiotics
IIIa	4 (15.4)	Obstruction of a double-J catheter with or without pyrexia	Catheter exchange
IIIb	0	–	–
IVa	0	–	–
IVb	1 (3.9)	Peritonitis due to urine leakage	Laparotomy
V	0	–	–

pyeloplasty (three sessions of extracorporeal shock wave lithotripsy) (Table 4).

The WHOQOL-BREF questionnaire demonstrated that patients evaluated the QoL as good (average 4 on 1–5 scale) and health condition as moderate (average 3.5 on 1–5 scale). Three (12.5%) patients were discontented with the health status (Table 5). Concerning the social domains in the WHOQOL-BREF questionnaire, the highest score was reported for the social relationship and lowest for physical health (Table 6).

4 Discussion

Minimally invasive pyeloplasty is the gold standard for the treatment of ureteropelvic junction obstruction. Clinical outcomes are excellent with the improvement observed in 85–100% of patients. Several surgical approaches appear equally effective (Janczak et al. 2018; Krajewski et al. 2017; Szydełko et al. 2012). The present study confirmed the good outcome of laparoscopic pyeloplasty as 88.5% of patients presented at the several-year long follow-up the correct urine passage from the renal pelvis into the ureter, which was confirmed by diuretic renography, and 80.8% of patients reported a reduction in painful urination.

Three of our patients did not have furosemide half-clearance time reduced to below 12 min. Each of them, despite not showing the expected outcome in diuretic renography, was satisfied with the pyeloplasty result, due likely to reduced

Table 3 Long-term follow-up outcomes after laparoscopic pyeloplasty in patients with ureteropelvic junction obstruction

Follow-up; mean ± SD (months)		89.8 ± 25.5
Age during control; mean ± SD, range (years)		39.3 ± 10.2 (21–64)
T½ - halftime to tracer clearance in diuretic renography; n (%), mean ± SD (min)	< 12 min	23 (88.5), 5.6 ± 2.3
	> 12 < 20 min	2 (7.7), 12.8 ± 1.0
	≥ 20 min	1 (3.9)
T½; depending on the presence of crossing vessels (CV); n (%), mean ± SD (min)	CV present	12 (46.2), 4.7 ± 4.1
	CV absent	14 (53.8), 6.0 ± 2.6
Hydronephrosis found in ultrasonography; n (%)	Absent	8 (29.6)
	Grade 1–2	11 (42.3)
	Grade 3–4	7 (26.9)
	Mean/median antero-posterior pelvis diameter (mm)	20.7/16.4
VAS (mean ± SD) (points)	Preoperative	6.4 ± 3.5
	Postoperative	1.4 ± 1.7
VAS reduction; n (%), mean ± SD (points)	Severe-to-mild	18 (69.2), (VAS from 7.6 ± 1.2 to 1.2 ± 1.2) p = 0.02
	Moderate-to-mild	3 (11.5), (VAS from 7.3 ± 0.6 to 3.0 ± 1.0) p = 0.04
	Severe-to-moderate	2 (7.7), (VAS from 8.5 ± 0.7 to 5.0 ± 1.4) p = 0.09
	Asymptomatic patients	3 (11.5%), (VAS from 0 to 0)

VAS visual analog scale of pain

Table 4 Results of own survey questionnaire for health-related quality of life

Are you satisfied with the pyeloplasty outcome?	Yes	25 (96.2%)
	No	1 (3.9%)
Would you agree to have another laparoscopic pyeloplasty if needed?	Yes	25 (96.2%)
	No	1 (3.9%)
How do you estimate your present intensity of the pain (points)	1.4 ± 1.7	
Does the pain significantly affect your life and professional activity?	Significantly	0
	Insignificantly	4 (15.4%)
	Not at all	22 (84.6%)
How many additional procedures did you undergo due to complications after pyeloplasty?	Antibiotic or antipyretic administration	3 patients
	Change of double-J catheter	4 patients
	Laparotomy	1 patient
	ESWL	1 patient

VAS visual analog scale of pain, *ESWL* extracorporeal shock wave lithotripsy

pain intensity when voiding. Nonetheless, they had to remain under close observation. Good clinical outcome, with the furosemide half-clearance time below 12 min and pain reduction, was also noticed in 18 patients with postoperative kidney hydronephrosis. Interestingly, a single patient who reported dissatisfaction with pyeloplasty due to an insufficient reduction in pain intensity did have the furosemide half-clearance time below 12 min and no kidney

Table 5 General subjective quality of life (QoL) and health status (HS) based on the World Health Organization Quality of Life (WHOQOL-BREF) questionnaire

Quality of Life			Health status	
Score	Patients (n)	%	Patients (n)	%
1	0	0	0	0
2	0	0	3	12.5%
3	4	16.7%	6	25.0%
4	16	66.7%	14	58.3%
5	4	16.7%	1	4.2%

Table 6 Domains of the World Health Organization Quality of Life (WHOQOL-BREF) questionnaire

	Score
Domain	Mean ± SD (range)
Physical health	54.1 ± 9.4 (38–69)
Psychological	68.0 ± 10.3 (44–88)
Social relationship	77.4 ± 9.4 (69–100)
Environment	65.8 ± 9.4 (44–81)

hydronephrosis. Likewise, most patients with other complications noted on the Clavien-Dindo grading scale reported a substantial pain reduction when voiding, satisfying QoL, and would agree to have another pyeloplasty procedure if needed.

The WHOQOL-BREF score in the health domain, somehow discrepantly, lagged the excellent surgical outcome of pyeloplasty. It reached an average of 3.5 points on the 1–5 scale, even though the global QoL score was better, reaching 4 points. A poorer perception of health could be influenced by comorbidities, which was not controlled for in the present study. Sahai et al. (2007) have shown a lack of difference between preoperative and postoperative physical QoL among patients who underwent laparoscopic upper urinary tract surgery for non-malignant conditions. However, there was a significant improvement in the postoperative mental QoL caused by relief from the emotional stress associated with pending surgery. Pace et al. (2003), comparing the effects of open and laparoscopic nephrectomy, have found that QoL one-year postoperatively returns to the baseline value faster in the laparoscopy-treated patients. In the present study, postoperative QoL was assessed at least 5 years after laparoscopy. Thus, it is a reasonable assumption that the patient's bias caused by perioperative stress and pain is negligible.

This study has several limitations. Data regarding preoperative and early postoperative periods were gathered retrospectively. The sample size was not big enough to perform a telling multifactorial analysis of factors affecting the QoL, concerning, for instance, the effects of surgical modifications or the presence of crossing vessels on the QoL. A low recruitment rate (26 out of the 95 patients invited to participate) could be caused by the fact that our clinic is one of a few reference centers in Poland performing laparoscopic pyeloplasty. Patients often come from distant locations, which limits their ability to participate. Additionally, a lack of symptoms in young adults, most patients were 30 years of age, makes them reluctant to undergo control tests. It seems unlikely that a low participation rate could result from poor surgery outcomes, considering a high success rate of laparoscopic pyeloplasty showed in this study. On the other hand, a success rate could introduce a "satisfaction" bias consisting of the greater willingness to participate in those patients who were satisfied when compared to dissatisfied, which could not be controlled for. Finally, the health-related QoL questionnaires were given to patients at the follow-up visit only.

Despite the limitations above outlined, we believe we have shown that patients suffering from ureteropelvic junction obstruction have a good clinical outcome associated with painful urination as well as psychological outcome concerning satisfaction with treatment results and quality of life at the long-term follow-up after laparoscopic pyeloplasty. The findings of this study may encourage both urological surgeons and patients in the decision-making for laparoscopic pyeloplasty to treat ureteropelvic junction obstruction.

Conflicts of Interest The authors of this manuscript have no conflicts of interest to disclose concerning this article.

Ethical Approval All procedures performed in studies involving human participants complied with the ethical standards of the institutional and/or national research committee and with the 1964 Helsinki declaration and its later amendments or comparable ethical standards. The study was approved by the Bioethics Committee of Wroclaw Medical University in Wrocląw, Poland; permit nr KB-458/2012.

Informed Consent All patients gave informed consent to participate in the study.

References

Autorino R, Eden C, El-Ghoneimi A, Guazzoni G, Buffi N, Peters CA, Stein RJ, Gettman M (2014) Robot-assisted and laparoscopic repair of ureteropelvic junction obstruction: a systematic review and meta-analysis. Eur Urol 65(2):430–452

Dindo D, Demartines N, Clavien PA (2004) Classification of surgical complications: a new proposal with evaluation in a cohort of 6336 patients and results of a survey. Ann Surg 240(2):205–213

García-Aparicio L, Blazquez-Gomez E, Martin O, Manzanares A, García-Smith N, Bejarano M, Rodo J, Ribó JM (2014) Anderson-Hynes pyeloplasty in patients less than 12 months old. Is the laparoscopic approach safe and feasible? J Endourol 28(8):906–908

Hawker GA, Mian S, Kendzerska T, French M (2011) Measures of adult pain: Visual Analog Scale for Pain (VAS Pain), Numeric Rating Scale for Pain (NRS Pain), McGill Pain Questionnaire (MPQ), Short-Form McGill Pain Questionnaire (SF-MPQ), Chronic Pain Grade Scale (CPGS), Short Form-36 Bodily Pain Scale (SF-36 BPS), and measure of Intermittent and Constant Osteoarthritis Pain (ICOAP). Arthritis Care Res 63 (Suppl 11):S240–S252

Janczak D, Szydełko U, Apoznański W, Panek W, Szydełko T (2018) W-type suture in Anderson-Hynes laparoscopic pyeloplasty: a novel approach to an old technique. Wideochir Inne Tech Maloinwazyjne 13 (4):512–517

Kavoussi LR, Peters CA (1993) Laparoscopic pyeloplasty. J Urol 150(6):1891–1894

Khoder WY, Waidelich R, Becker AJ, Karl A, Haseke N, Bauer RM, Stief CG, Bachmann A, Ebinger Mundorff N (2014) Patients' perception of surgical outcomes and quality of life after retroperitoneoscopic and open pyeloplasty. Urol Int 92(1):74–82

Knoedler J, Han L, Granberg C, Kramer S, Chow G, Gettman M, Kimball B, Moriarty J, Kim S, Husmann D (2013) Population-based comparison of laparoscopic and open pyeloplasty in pediatric pelvi-ureretic junction obstruction. BJU Int 111(7):1141–1147

Krajewski W, Wojciechowska J, Dembowski J, Zdrojowy R, Szydełko T (2017) Hydronephrosis in the course of ureteropelvic junction obstruction: an underestimated problem? Current opinions on the pathogenesis, diagnosis and treatment. Adv Clin Exp Med 26(5):857–864

Pace KT, Dyer SJ, Stewart RJ, Honey RJ, Poulin EC, Schlachta CM, Mamazza J (2003) Health-related quality of life after laparoscopic and open nephrectomy. Surg Endosc 17(1):143–152

Panek W, De Jong TPVM, Szydełko T, Chrzan R (2019) Management of crossing vessels in children and adults: a multi–center experience with the transperitoneal laparoscopic approach. Adv Clin Exp Med 28 (6):777–782

Parekh AD, Thomas JC, Trusler L, Ankerst DP, Deshpande JK, Adams MC, Pope JC 4th, Brock JW 3rd (2008) Prospective evaluation of health related quality of life for pediatric patients with ureteropelvic junction obstruction. J Urol 180(5):2171–2176

Sahai A, Tang S, Challacombe B, Murphy D, Dasgupta P (2007) Laparoscopic upper urinary tract surgery for benign and malignant conditions. Does etiology have an effect on health-related quality of life? Int J Clin Pract 61(12):2026–2029

Schuessler WW, Grune MT, Tecuanhuey LV, Preminger GM (1993) Laparoscopic dismembered pyeloplasty. J Urol 150(6):1795–1799

Strother MC, Mucksavage P (2016) Minimally invasive techniques for the management of adult UPJ obstruction. Curr Urol Rep 17(5):39

Szydełko T, Kasprzak J, Apoznański W, Kołodziej A, Zdrojowy R, Dembowski J, Niezgoda T (2010) Comparison of dismembered and nondismembered Y-V laparoscopic pyeloplasty in patients with primary hydronephrosis. J Laparoendosc Adv Surg Tech 20 (1):7–12

Szydełko T, Kasprzak J, Lewandowski J, Apoznański W, Dembowski J (2012) Dismembered laparoscopic Anderson-Hynes pyeloplasty versus nondismembered laparoscopic Y-V pyeloplasty in the treatment of patients with primary ureteropelvic junction obstruction: a prospective study. J Endourol 26(9):1165–1170

Adv Exp Med Biol - Clinical and Experimental Biomedicine (2022) 13: 53–62
https://doi.org/10.1007/5584_2021_631

Published online: 3 April 2021

Causes and Effects of Introducing Surgery Safety Checklist: A Review

Jacek Lorkowski, Izabella Maciejowska-Wilcock, and Mieczysław Pokorski

Abstract

The medical treatment process, particularly surgery, is inescapably bound to potential complications or undesirable adverse events. This narrative review aims to present the causes and effects of the introduction of the WHO Surgery Safety Checklist (SSC), the use of which is expected to reduce the number of perioperative errors, complications, and mortality. To achieve this objective, we performed a bibliometric analysis of medical citations indexed in the PubMed database using the SSC subject heading. Findings revealed a total of 1441 articles meeting inclusion status, with 1171 published during the last decade. After the screening of titles and abstracts, the members of the research team selected 75 articles, deemed most relevant for inclusion in the review, which were then thoroughly analyzed. All in all, the findings were that the use of SSC appreciably reduced the number of simple logistic errors in the perioperative period decreasing the frequency of resulting complications and mortality.

Keywords

Adverse effects · Mortality · Perioperative complications · Surgery safety checklist

1 Introduction

The treatment process, particularly surgery, is inescapably bound to potential errors and complications that may have a substantial bearing on outcome inclusive of fatality. Identifying the causes of such events, including death in the operating theater, is a difficult task. Most studies focus on risk factors resulting from the pathophysiological mechanisms of diseases. To substantiate the relationship to erroneous human activity is a challenge (Vincent et al. 2004). Nonetheless, difficult to explain undesirable events is most often attributed to medical staff (El Bardissi and Sundt 2012). To improve patient safety, the American Institute of Medicine and the National Academy of Engineering promoted the use of techniques tailored to assist the human factor. Tools were

J. Lorkowski (✉)
Department of Orthopedics, Traumatology and Sports Medicine, Central Clinical Hospital of the Ministry of Internal Affairs and Administration, Warsaw, Poland

Faculty of Health Sciences, Medical University of Mazovia, Warsaw, Poland
e-mail: jacek.lorkowski@gmail.com

I. Maciejowska-Wilcock
Jagiellonian Language Center of the Jagiellonian University, Cracow, Poland
e-mail: izabella.maciejowska@uj.edu.pl

M. Pokorski
Institute of Health Sciences, Opole University, Opole, Poland

Faculty of Health Sciences, The Jan Długosz University in Częstochowa, Częstochowa, Poland
e-mail: m.pokorski@ujd.edu.pl

developed to improve and optimize the safety of medical activities (Boillat et al. 2019). Recent research shows that most often errors do not result from the actions of individuals but conflicting, incomplete, or suboptimal systems. The concept of the system is broad. It covers all logistic activities of people, technologies, equipment, materials, and the environment in which they occur (Carayon et al. 2006).

Multidisciplinary analyses indicate that the most common cause of adverse events in healthcare lies in the transmission of information that may be delivered incompletely, not at all, or to the wrong person. Further, problems existing for many years often remain unsolved until a crisis occurs (Zavalkoff et al. 2011). All these factors were considered by the WHO while developing guidelines for procedures necessary for patient safety, notably including patients subjected to surgery (WHO 2009). The guidelines took the form of the surgery safety checklist (SSC), a 19-item tool created in association with the Harvard School of Public Health in June 2008. This review aims to present the effects of the introduction of SSC on the number of perioperative complications and mortality. To achieve this objective, we performed a bibliometric analysis of medical citations indexed in the PubMed database as of November 2020 using the "surgery safety checklist" as the subject heading. We revealed a total of 1441 articles meeting inclusion status, 1327 of which were full-text publications. There were 1171 articles dated in the last decade. Among them, there were 54 clinical trials and 231 review articles. The members of the research team screened the titles and abstracts of 811 articles of the last decade and selected 75 of them, deemed most relevant, which were thoroughly analyzed for inclusion in the review.

2 Reasons for Introducing the Surgery Safety Checklist (SSC)

The WHO conducted large-scale research on the outcomes of surgical treatment. The preliminary results became known at the beginning of the twenty-first century. The findings are that perioperative mortality in patients undergoing major surgical procedures in industrialized countries is low (0.01%) (Braz et al. 2009), but the prevalence of significant undesirable events and complications reaches an alarming proportion of 3–16% (Weiser et al. 2008). These complications could have been preventable in one-half of the cases. For comparison, the most underdeveloped countries of Sub-Saharan Africa grapple with the mortality of 0.67% in patients during general anesthesia. African countries also lead in perioperative complications due to a shortage of licensed medical staff, equipment, and medicines, as well as the combination of simple organizational mistakes or unfavorable factors that should never happen. For instance, communication and teamwork issues are responsible for as many as 70% of undesirable events in obstetrics (Ogunlusi et al. 2017; Nwosu 2015; De Vries et al. 2008).

According to the estimations of independent authors as well as governmental agencies or WHO, 234 M surgical operations are performed annually in the world. Presuming a 10% perioperative rate of significant undesirable events, the issue comes down to the population exceeding one-half of the average European country, like Poland. Concerning fatalities, the number comes to about 1 M, globally, in the periprocedural or postoperative period (Weiser et al. 2008; WHO 2008a). The socioeconomic impact of this number of undesirable events is enormous. The important factor is, however, that a large proportion, reaching one-half of complications, could have been avoided. Numerous researchers, including WHO experts, indicate the possibility of a significant reduction in the number of errors made, using the simplest methods strengthening the hygienic and organizational milieu of operative theaters. An outstandingly high rate of perioperative complication and mortality in Sub-Saharan countries above outlined was one factor behind the introduction of the WHO SSC. A notorious shortage of qualified medical personnel compounds the issue (Collins et al. 2014; Vivekanantham et al. 2014). In the 2000s, WHO estimated the global shortage of health workers at

4.2 M, with 1 M new workers needed immediately in Sub-Saharan Africa alone (Crisp et al. 2008; Chen et al. 2004). Of the 64 selected hospitals in East Africa, only 4% had an adequately trained anesthesiologist, 92% had one anesthesia nurse at the most, and 8% had "anesthesia assistants" who substituted for trained anesthsiologists and were able to manage only a few selected procedures. The hospitals had to ask for help from neighboring ones. It was only in the last 10 years in Uganda, a country of about 40 M, that the number of anesthesiologists increased from 13 to 50, who work mainly in large urban areas (Hodges et al. 2007). Besides, the priority was to ensure safe anesthesia during delivery and C-sections, which is in line with WHO recommendations (Epiu et al. 2016). Concurrently, anesthesia standards have been worked out and published to be applied not only in tertiary hospitals but also in referral hospitals where medical care is provided for the largest chunk of the population (Epiu et al. 2017b). Similar studies and analyses were conducted in five national hospitals of the highest reference level in East Africa in Uganda, Kenya, Tanzania, Rwanda, and Burundi. Disappointingly, it has been found that none meets all the World Federation of Societies of Anaesthesiologists (WFSA) requirements for ensuring safe obstetric anesthesia (Epiu et al. 2017a). Anesthesia requires the presence of a doctor. The mere availability of the equipment is not enough. This is due to the need for comprehensive knowledge of the physiology and understanding of the anesthetic process itself. The doctor is necessary to ensure the safety of the entire anesthesia process, particularly the patency of airways, and to cope with hypo- or hyperventilation (Enright and Merry 2009). A 2016 review has reported that anesthesia contributes to 13.8% of all maternal deaths following C-sections. The mortality is almost twice as often when anesthesia is performed by non-anesthesiologists. Of all deaths, 76% results from complications in the respiratory tract, while the remaining cases are due to the employee's incompetence or logistic errors (Sobhy et al. 2016). Challenges faced by anesthesiologists and surgeons in many low-income countries include working in underinvested hospitals and shortages of staff, trained anesthesiologists and surgeons, equipment, materials, and often essential medications (Melekie and Getahun 2015; Grimes et al. 2011). A combination of unfavorable factors and the overwrought surgical and anesthetic teams lead to an increase in the prosaic medical errors (Collins et al. 2014; Vivekanantham et al. 2014). With the existing shortages and deficiencies, more complex cases must be treated in larger centers, which leads to excessive workload there and becomes another potential cause of adverse events (Barnes-Josiah et al. 1998).

In synopsis, doctors working in the countries of Sub-Saharan Africa face a significant shortage of equipment, particularly necessary for safe anesthesia. That applies to both surgery and childbirth. The problem is amplified by a shortage of staff necessary to ensure effective perioperative care. Additionally, shortages in these countries also concern trained and competent suppliers of equipment and service thereof. Therefore, key resources ensuring safe healthcare are missing. Reports indicate that only 5% of hospitals meet the requirements for operating and recovery rooms set by the World Federation of Societies of Anaesthesiologists (WFSA). Attention has also been directed to significant shortages of blood and blood products necessary for the safe conduct of procedures (Epiu et al. 2016). The issues outlined above have been the background for the introduction of the SSC.

Problem-solving efforts in the first place involve the implementation of the simplest solutions that do not require large financial outlays. It has been assumed that the introduction and obligatory use of a specific checklist would help put procedures on halt in case of shortages of staff and equipment, or ambiguities concerning the place and type of surgery. Due to the existing shortage of physicians in Africa, the focus was put on the training of non-physician staff who could take over the role of SSC coordinators and supervisors. Such a person should acquire the formal qualifications and skills of a group leader and be empowered to halt ongoing procedures, e.g., stop the surgery. Incidentally, women turned out to be the most suitable candidates for this role from a psychophysiological standpoint. That, however, has required a turn-around in the hitherto stereotypical mental attitude of African people where men distinctly predominate in professional activities (WHO 2008b). Currently, many training programs improve patient safety and, simultaneously, develop leadership skills (Weaver et al. 2013). These activities vary by country and hospital, but some elements are common such as training by hospital board members and managers, or by healthcare risk leaders concerning the patient's safety (Schwendimann et al. 2013; Frankel et al. 2008; Thomas et al. 2005).

3 Principles of Surgery Safety Checklist (SSC)

The guiding principle of SSC is to help improve communication within the team and shape teamwork, reduce the number of perioperative errors and complications, and thus improve the patient's safety and treatment outcome. The WHO, introducing the SSC, outlined ten basic goals of safe surgery. Based on them, a 19-point questionnaire was created which systematizes verification procedures. Three stages of SSC use were distinguished. The first one refers to the time before the induction of anesthesia, the second before the first incision, and the third before the patient leaves the operating theater. Recommendations for the first stage are as follows: verification of the patient's identity, confirmation of consent to the surgery, confirmation of the place and type of the planned surgical procedure, confirmation of the airway assessment, and the inspection of equipment. The second stage consists of the confirmation of individual roles in the procedure, analysis of possible emergencies, surgery duration, and antibiotic prophylaxis. The final stage concerns the procedures related to the way the patient leaves the operating theater. During or immediately after wound closure, before the patient is taken away, the remaining surgical supplies and equipment must be checked to ensure nothing is left behind, results of any intraoperative examinations archived, and basic postoperative recommendations set forward. The introduction of SSC has been associated with a reduction in operational errors and lower rates of undesirable events worldwide, including low and middle-income countries (DeMaria and Neustein 2010; Seiden and Barach 2006; Gibbs 2005). The introduction and success of SSC are liable to stem from the psychological aptitude to follow imposed recommendations, making the staff act accordingly. For instance, as Epiu et al. (2016) have noted, over a century-old recommendation "wash your hands with soap" resulted in a dramatic drop in the perioperative infection rate. Contemporary estimates are that the implementation of SSC helped avoid eight deaths and save about $ 2 M in healthcare costs in just one hospital.

4 Knowledge and Effects of Surgery Safety Checklist (SSC)

As is the case with any tool, employees must be aware of its existence to use it. The WHO has put a lot of effort into spreading the knowledge about the existence of SSC (WHO 2008b). At present, the SSC is well known and widely used not only among specialists in the USA and EU but also in other countries of the world (Epiu et al. 2017a, b; Epiu et al. 2016; Sobhy et al. 2016; Melekie and Getahun 2015; Grimes et al. 2011; DeMaria and Neustein 2010). Even in a rather distant from the mainstream surgery field of dental implantology at the School of Dental Medicine of the University of Connecticut, the SSC has been familiarized with, implemented, and its usefulness in the prevention of perioperative threats presented in a special promotion program (Remiszewski and Bidra 2019). Surveys conducted in Africa and South and Central Americas show that SSC is well known as its existence has been confirmed by over 90% of respondents (Ogunlusi et al. 2017; Haynes et al. 2011).

According to the literature, the most common reaction to SSC among medical staff is a positive attitude (93%) following the initial hesitation (Vivekanantham et al. 2014). It is believed that the SSC increases the interest in the issue of perioperative patient safety (Sucupira et al. 2016). Research conducted in Finland, which is a representative reflection of the whole of Scandinavia, shows that the implementation of SSC significantly increases the awareness of surgical teams in this regard, leading to the revisions of procedures in place and possible threats (Takala et al. 2011). Another approach, often encountered in underdeveloped countries, may be exemplified by Nigeria where about 93% of respondents know about the usefulness of SSC but are dissatisfied with the insufficient use of its recommendations in hospitals (Ogunlusi et al. 2017).

The authors dealing with the SSC issues focus on communication and interpersonal cooperation within the multidisciplinary surgical-anesthetic team. In principle, a team is a group of professionals united by one basic goal, which is the patient safety and optimal performance of the procedure. The overwhelming majority of respondents find that the SSC is conducive to intra-team communication (Santana et al. 2016; Russ et al. 2015; McDowell and McComb 2014; Berrisford et al. 2012; De Vries et al. 2011; Kearns et al. 2011; W-Dahl et al. 2011; Abdel-Galil 2010). An integrated team is gradually formed, engaged in joint work. This is achieved by training, which is particularly important for the originally disintegrated group of people (Melekie and Getahun 2015).

5 Implementation of Surgery Safety Checklist (SSC)

The way the hospital management implements the SSC procedures varies. At one extreme, there is the institutional compulsion and pointing to the obligations resulting from the employment contract, and at the other, the issue may be downplayed (Bosk et al. 2009; Hales and Pronovost 2006). At any rate, filling out the SSC documentation takes no more than 3–5 min, causing no distraction from the predefined duties (Russ et al. 2013). The implementation of SSC, like any other novelty, may cause some reluctance, particularly that new protocols are most often seen by medical staff as an increase in the number of a pile of existing duties. High routine uses of SSC, reaching 86%, takes place in university hospitals, which may result from a better organization of appropriate training and a more positive attitude of clinicians to new products (Vivekanantham et al. 2014). Non-university centers, particularly hospitals in the rural areas inhabited by low-income populations, face challenges such as an overload of patients and staff and equipment shortages, the circumstances that do not facilitate the use of SSC. However, SSC increases the probability of eliminating logistic errors in such conditions, so that it is essential healthcare professionals knowingly use it (Conley et al. 2011).

According to Ogunlusi et al. (2017), SSC is useful and lives up to its expectations in both developed and developing countries. A progressively increasing number of surgical procedures in developing countries have directed attention to strategies improving patient safety, particularly, when key resources like the availability of qualified medical staff are limited. The professional experience is still small there as only 68% of staff work in the hospital for less than 5 years. A survey performed among several dozens of surgeons, anesthesiologists, and operating theater nurses in Nigeria shows that 83% of them confirm knowledge of SSC. Among the respondents, however, only about 22% correctly states that the main purpose of SSC is to ensure patient safety by, inter alia, proper conduct of surgery. This shows that the reported over 80% knowledge of SSC is based on false assumptions as it is unlikely that the surveyed staff has comprehended the SSC sense. The main difficulties in the optimal use of SSC indicated by the respondents are the lack of training (58%), staff assertiveness (58%), and the inability to complete the paperwork in the required time frame (47%). These results show that more training and education on the use of SSC are necessary. A study performed in Ethiopia has shown that in about 40% of cases, SSC enters the mandatory use after a short basic training which is not followed up (Melekie and Getahun 2015). Likewise, Sewell et al. (2011) have shown the lack of training lies at the heart of non-use or misuse of SSC in more than one-half of instances. Joy et al. (2011) have shown that training in SSC conducted in classrooms and simulator laboratories increases the use of recommended algorithms and contributes to better treatment outcomes. Nonetheless, surgical teams often resist participating in such activities. Changing the organizational culture of the operating theater team appears a challenging endeavor. The logistic issue that should be solved during training is the elimination or shortening of unnecessary time breaks and delays that affect the number of surgical treatments by improving non-technical skills in the operating theater. It is necessary to adjust these activities allocating them to specific teams, where some staff has been working and cooperating for many years and some appear and disappear after a short while. Other authors indicate a need for conducting regular audits of problems related to the use of SSC and providing constructive feedback on an ongoing basis, which should be based on coaching rather than typical regular checks. The emphasis is put on a stress-free continuous training (Hancorn and Blair 2010; Birkmeyer and Miller 2009; Haynes et al. 2009).

6 Surgery Safety Checklist (SSC) and Treatment Outcomes

The reports show surgical treatment outcomes and patient safety have improved after the introduction of SSC (Santana et al. 2016; Mayer et al. 2015; McDowell and McComb 2014; Kearns et al. 2011; Abdel-Galil 2010; DeMaria and Neustein 2010), with a clear decline in undesirable events. For instance, in Tunisia, a country with a modest income and work culture hardly compatible with the Anglo-Saxon standards, the eyebrow-raising 60% of undesirable events have been prevented by using the SSC as reported in a large retrospective study (Letaief et al. 2010). The most frightful undesirable event is death. A survey performed in the South Carolina hospitals has shown a reduction in the number of surgery-related deaths in the first 3 years after the implementation and completion of the SSC-based quality improvement program when compared with hospitals that do not use such algorithms. This also speaks for the increased patient safety while using the SSC (Haynes et al. 2017). The most informative studies show that the correct systematic use of SSC reduces the number of complications and mortality from 19.9% to 11.5% and 1.6% to 1.0%, respectively (Haugen et al. 2015; Haynes et al. 2009). The improvement in outcomes has been also shown in Scottish hospitals participating in the Patient Safety Program (SPSP) assessing the emergency surgeries performed in 2000-2014. The assessment concerned a cohort of 6,839,736 patients who were operated on, out of the 12,667,926 admitted to hospitals. A distinct overall decline in a surgical mortality rate of 36.6% was noted in surgical patients, remaining unchanged in non-surgical ones, since the implementation of SSC, with the annual mortality rate decreasing by 0.003% and 0.069% before versus after implementation, respectively (Ramsay et al. 2019).

A large study on the clinical role of SSC was also performed in a culturally different environment in China. The analysis covered 7209 patients with gastrointestinal cancer who underwent elective surgery at the Affiliated Hospital of Qingdao University. Data on patients who underwent surgery before the introduction of SSC were gathered retrospectively (3238 consecutive surgeries) and prospectively in those treated after its introduction (3971 surgeries). The incidence of complications, in-hospital mortality, and the median hospitalization duration before and after the SSC introduction, the latter verified by mandatory SSC documentation, were 16.4% versus 14.3%, 0.46% versus 0.18%, and 9 versus 8 days, respectively. Multivariate analysis shows the SSC was an independent factor decreasing the number of postoperative complications (odds ratio = 0.86; 95% confidence intervals 0.75-0.99) and thus, improving surgical outcome in gastrointestinal cancer (Wang et al. 2019). Likewise, other studies have also reported that the introduction of SSC or other checklists is associated with a reduction in postoperative complications (De Vries et al. 2010; Vats et al. 2010; Edmondson et al. 2001). The use of SSC is particularly useful in "acute" cases and in situations requiring improvisation when there is the greatest probability of potential mistakes (Melekie and Getahun 2015). Additionally, the SSC helps avoid the confusion the patients may experience concerning the time and site of the planned surgery. A Guatemalan study has shown that the use of SSC decreases the chance of performing a mistaken procedure in the wrong patient (Ogunlusi et al. 2017; Ragusa et al. 2016). Unfortunately, despite more than 10 years of campaigning to prevent the happening of such erroneous events, they continue to crop up. Performing the wrong surgery or on the wrong body side still takes occasionally place.

Strangely enough, authors from France and the UK, where the SSC is mandatory, report the average number of correctly completed SSC documents is only 60% (Boillat et al. 2019; Fourcade et al. 2011; Warnock 2010). This finding seems a more complex and common issue concerning more countries than these two. Russ et al. (2013) have reported in their review that 50% of respondents do not fully follow the algorithms that are part of SSC, which means the documents are not completed or procedures required before the patient leaves the operating theater are not fulfilled. For instance, surveys conducted among Nigerian anesthesiologists, where the response rate was 83.6%, indicated the use of SSC by 62.7% of respondents, mainly in university hospitals (86.2% vs. 23.3% and 14.3% in other types of hospitals). Physicians who most often used SSC were aged 35-44 (approx. 71%) and the least often were over 55 years old (approx. 60%). Although the existence of SSC was known for 93.1% of respondents, a large proportion disbelieved that the algorithms may prevent errors and other undesirable events (Olatosi et al. 2018). Likewise, a Brazilian study has found that the use of SSC is widespread, reaching as much as 90.3% of surgeries, but almost in no case, the associated procedures would be fully done. Frighteningly, as many as 95.4% of surgeries were continued after errors in the implemented safety algorithms had been unraveled. The errors noticed concerned the timing of procedures to be performed and the continuation of activities despite the lack of key specialists. Further, the operating team did not actively implement the recommendations resulting from SSC which was treated just as another hassle to be completed (Almeida and Rodrigues 2019).

The negligence of safety practices increases the risks involved with surgery. This is supported by another Brazilian study involving 502 orthopedic physicians. The study found that about 41% of physicians had experienced an undesirable event such as performing surgery on the wrong patient or the wrong body side. As many as 25.6% of physicians indicated "misunderstanding" as the cause of a mishap. Despite that, as many as 35.5% of the surveyed physicians still failed to mark the body side for surgery before transporting the patient to the operating theater. All the research shows that such mistakes could be avoided by using SCC. While attempting to justify their misactions, physicians cited the lack of having savvy about all the features of SSC (65.3%) or training in this area (72.1%) (Motta Filho et al. 2013).

The implementation of SSC also appears of substantial help in counteracting surgery-related thromboembolic episodes. There are studies from various centers that confirm the effectiveness of SSC use in decreasing the clinical burden of these all too often happening and sometimes fatal episodes (Berrisford et al. 2012; W-Dahl et al. 2011). One other issue often discussed is the role of SSC in perioperative antibiotic prophylaxis. An important piece of work on the matter is a comparative analysis of the effects of using SSC during surgical procedures performed on the large intestine in two economically and culturally different countries; Canada and Brazil. The implementation of SSC algorithms was compared to the lack thereof considering the rate of surgical site infections. It decreased by a few percentage points in both countries. The authors emphasize the unequivocal benefit of implementing the SSC, with relatively low financial outlays (Gama et al. 2019). A reduction in the rate of perioperative infections using the SSC standards has been also noticed in the investigation of other types of surgical procedures (Melekie and Getahun 2015; Boaz et al. 2014; De Vries et al. 2011; Haynes et al. 2011). Nonetheless, the success of antibiotic perioperative prophylaxis also depends, to a sizable extent, on specific hospital policies run by the specialized infection council or clinical bacteriologists, which usually differ by country and region. Antibiotic prophylaxis is adapted according to the microbial surveillance and the identification of pathogenic bacterial contaminants, and other local factors, all of which may go beyond and above simple compliance with the SSC algorithms. Therefore, antibiotic perioperative prophylaxis is a multifaceted process, the SSC is a major but unlikely a unique element of it (Siddiqi et al. 2019; Wæhle et al. 2019; Loozen et al. 2017; Vila et al. 2017).

In conclusion, the use of the WHO Surgery Safety Checklist, according to the overwhelming research, reduces the number of simple logistic errors in the perioperative period, thereby also error-related complications and mortality rate in surgical patients.

Conflict of Interest The authors declare no conflict of interest concerning this article.

Ethical Approval This review article does not contain any studies with human participants or animals performed by any of the authors.

References

Abdel-Galil K (2010) The WHO surgical safety checklist: are we measuring up? Br J Oral Maxillofac Surg 48:397–498

Almeida RE, Rodrigues MCS (2019) Implementation of the surgical safety checklist for pediatric operations: compliance assessment. Rev Gaucha Enferm 40(spe): e20180270

Barnes-Josiah D, Myntti C, Augustin A (1998) The three delays, as a framework for examining maternal mortality in Haiti. Soc Sci Med 46(8):981–993

Berrisford RG, Wilson IH, Davidge M, Sanders D (2012) Surgical time out checklist with debriefing and multidisciplinary feedback improves venous thromboembolism prophylaxis in thoracic surgery: a prospective audit. Eur J Cardiothorac Surg 41(6):1326–1329

Birkmeyer JD, Miller DC (2009) Surgery: can checklists improve surgical outcomes? Nat Rev Urol 6:245–246

Boaz M, Bermant A, Ezri T, Lakstein D, Berlovitz Y, Laniado I, Feldbrin Z (2014) Effect of Surgical Safety checklist implementation on the occurrence of postoperative complications in orthopedic patients. Isr Med Assoc J 16(1):20–25

Boillat T, Grantcharov P, Rivas H (2019) Increasing completion rate and benefits of checklists: prospective evaluation of surgical safety checklists with smart glasses. JMIR Mhealth Uhealth 7(4):e13447

Bosk CL, Dixon-Woods M, Goeschel CA, Goeschel CA, Pronovost PJ (2009) Perspective: reality checks for checklists. Lancet 374(9688):444–445

Braz LG, Braz DG, da Cruz DS, Fernandes LA, Módolo NSP, Braz JRC (2009) Mortality in anesthesia: a systematic review. Clinics (Sao Paulo) 64(10):999–1006

Carayon P, Schoofs HA, Karsh B, Gurses AP, Alvarado CJ, Smith M, Flatley Brennan P (2006) Work system design for patient safety: the SEIPS model. Qual Saf Health Care 15(Suppl 1):I50–I58

Chen L, Evans T, Anand S, Boufford JI, Brown H, Chowdhury M, Cueto M, Dare L, Dussault G, Elzinga G, Fee E, Habte D, Hanvoravongchai P, Jacobs M, Kurowski C, Michael S, Pablos-Mendez A, Sewankambo N, Solimano G, Stilwell B, de Waal A, Wibulpolprasert S (2004) Human resources for health: overcoming the crisis. Lancet 364(9449):1984–1990

Collins SJ, Newhouse R, Porter J, Talsma A (2014) Effectiveness of the surgical safety checklist in correcting errors: a literature review applying Reason's Swiss cheese model. AORN J 100:65–779.e5

Conley DM, Singer SJ, Edmondson L, Berry WR, Gawande AA (2011) Effective surgical safety checklist implementation. J Am Coll Surg 212(5):873–879

Crisp N, Gawanas B, Sharp I, Task Force for Scaling Up Education and Training for Health Workers (2008) Training the health workforce: scaling up, saving lives. Lancet 371(9613):689–691

DeMaria S Jr, Neustein SM (2010) Production pressure, medical errors, and the pre-anesthesia checkout. Middle East J Anaesthesiol 20:631–638

De Vries EN, Boermeester MA, Gouma DJ (2008) WHO's checklist for surgery: don't confine it to the operating room. Lancet 372(9644):1148–1149

De Vries EN, Eikens-Jansen MP, Hamersma AM, Smorenburg SM, Gouma DJ, Boermeester MA (2011) Prevention of surgical malpractice claims by use of a surgical safety checklist. Ann Surg 253:624–628

De Vries EN, Prins HA, Crolla RM, den Outer AJ, van Andel G, van Helden SH, Schlack WS, van Putten MA, Gouma DJ, Dijkgraaf MG, Smorenburg SM, SURPASS Collaborative Group (2010) Effect of a comprehensive surgical safety system on patient outcomes. N Engl J Med 363:1963–1965

Edmondson AC, Bohmer RM, Pisano GP (2001) Disrupted routines: team learning and new technology implementation in hospitals. Adm Sci Q 46:685–716

El Bardissi AW, Sundt TM (2012) Human factors and operating room safety. Surg Clin North Am 92 (1):21–35

Enright A, Merry A (2009) The WFSA and patient safety in the perioperative setting. Can J Anesth 56(1):8–13

Epiu I, Mijumbi C, Chokwe T, Lugazia E, Twagirumugabe T, Ndarugire F, Tindimwebwa JVB, Dubowitz G (2017a) Challenges of anesthesia in low-and middle-income countries: a cross-sectional survey of access to safe obstetric anesthesia in East Africa. Anesth Analg 124(1):290–299

Epiu I, Tindimwebwa JV, Mijumbi C, Ndarugirire F, Twagirumugabe T, Lugazia ER, Dubowitz G, Chokwe TM (2016) Working towards safer surgery in Africa; a survey of utilization of the WHO safe surgical checklist at the main referral hospitals in East Africa. BMC Anesthesiol 16(1):60

Epiu I, Wabule A, Kambugu A, Mayanja-Kizza H, Tindimwebwa JVB, Dubowitz G (2017b) Key bottlenecks to the provision of safe obstetric anaesthesia in low-income countries; a cross-sectional survey of 64 hospitals in Uganda. BMC Pregnancy Childbirth 17 (1):387

Fourcade A, Blache J, Grenier C, Bourgain J, Minvielle E (2011) Barriers to staff adoption of a surgical safety checklist. BMJ Qual Saf 21(3):191–197

Frankel A, Grillo SP, Pittman M, Thomas EJ, Horowitz L, Page M, Sexton B (2008) Revealing and resolving patient safety defects the impact of leadership WalkRounds on frontline caregiver assessments of patient safety. Health Serv Res 43(6):2050–2066

Gama CS, Backman C, Oliveira AC (2019) Effect of surgical safety checklist on colorectal surgical site infection rates in 2 countries: Brazil and Canada. Am J Infect Control l47(9):1112–1117

Gibbs VC (2005) Patient safety practices in the operating room: correct-site surgery and nothing left behind. Surg Clin North Am 85:1307–1319

Grimes CE, Bowman KG, Dodgion CM, Lavy CB (2011) Systematic review of barriers to surgical care in low-income and middle-income countries. World J Surg 35(5):941–950

Hales BM, Pronovost PJ (2006) The checklist – a tool for error management and performance improvement. J Crit Care 21:231–235

Hancorn K, Blair S (2010) Checklist culture: who needs changing? BMJ 340:90–99

Haugen AS, Søfteland E, Almeland SK, Sevdalis N, Vonen B, Eide GE, Nortvedt MW, Harthug S (2015) Effect of the World Health Organization checklist on patient outcomes: a stepped wedge cluster randomized controlled trial. Ann Surg 261(5):821–828

Haynes AB, Edmondson L, Lipsitz SR, Molina G, Neville BA, Singer SJ, Moonan AT, Childers AK, Foster R, Gibbons LR, Gawande AA, Berry WR (2017) Mortality trends after a voluntary checklist-based surgical safety collaborative. Ann Surg 266(6):923–929

Haynes AB, Weiser TG, Berry WR, Lipsitz SR, Breizat AH, Dellinger EP, Dziekan G, Herbosa T, Kibatala PL, Lapitan MC, Merry AF, Reznick RK, Taylor B, Vats A, Gawande AA, Safe Surgery Saves Lives Study Group (2011) Changes in safety attitude and relationship to decreased postoperative morbidity and mortality following implementation of a checklist-based surgical safety intervention. Qual Saf Health Care 20(1):102–107

Haynes AB, Weiser TG, Berry WR, Lipsitz SR, Breizat AH, Dellinger EP, Herbosa T, Joseph S, Kibatala PL, Lapitan MC, Merry AF, Moorthy K, Reznick RK, Taylor B, Gawande AA (2009) A surgical safety checklist to reduce morbidity and mortality in a global population. N Engl J Med 360:491–499

Hodges SC, Mijumbi C, Okello M, McCormick BA, Walker IA, Wilson IH (2007) Anaesthesia services in developing countries: defining the problems. Anaesthesia 62(1):4–11

Joy BF, Elliott E, Hardy C, Sullivan C, Backer CL, Kane JM (2011) Standardized multidisciplinary protocol improves handover of cardiac surgery patients to the intensive care unit. Pediatr Crit Care Med 12:304–308

Kearns RJ, Uppal V, Bonner J, Robertson J, Daniel M, McGrady EM (2011) The introduction of a surgical safety checklist in a tertiary referral obstetric center. BMJ Qual Saf 20:818–822

Letaief M, El Mhamdi S, El-Asady R, Siddiqi S, Abdullatif A (2010) Adverse events in a Tunisian hospital: results of a retrospective cohort study. Int J Qual Health Care 22(5):380–385

Loozen CS, van Santvoort HC, van Geloven AAW, Nieuwenhuijzen GAP, de Reuver PR, Besselink MHG, Vlaminckx B, Kelder JC, Knibbe CAJ, Boerma D (2017) Perioperative antibiotic prophylaxis in the treatment of acute cholecystitis (PEANUTS II trial): study protocol for a randomized controlled trial. Trials 18(1):390

Mayer EK, Sevdalis N, Rout S, Caris J, Russ S, Mansell J, Davies R, Skapinakis P, Vincent C, Athanasiou T, Moorthy K, Darzi A (2015) Measuring variation in use of the WHO surgical safety checklist in the operating room: a multicenter prospective cross-sectional study. J Am Coll Surg 220:1–11

McDowell DS, McComb SA (2014) Safety checklist briefings: a systematic review of the literature. AORN J 99:125–137

Melekie TB, Getahun GM (2015) Compliance with surgical safety checklist completion in the operating room of University of Gondar Hospital, Northwest Ethiopia. BMC Res Notes 8:361

Motta Filho GDR, Neves da Silva LF, Ferracini AM, Bähr GL (2013) The WHO Surgical Safety Checklist: knowledge and use by Brazilian orthopedists. Rev Bras Ortop 48(6):554–562

Nwosu A (2015) The horror of wrong-site surgery continues: report of two cases in a regional trauma center in Nigeria. Patient Saf Surg 9(1):6

Ogunlusi JD, Yusuf MB, Ogunsuyi PS, Wuraola OK, Babalola WO, Oluwadiya KS, Ajogbasile OO (2017) Awareness and use of surgical checklist among theater users at Ekiti State University Teaching Hospital, Ado-Ekiti, Nigeria. Niger J Surg 23(2):134–137

Olatosi JO, Anaegbu NC, Adesida A (2018) Use of the World Health Organization surgical Safety Checklist by Nigerian anesthetists. Niger J Surg 24(2):111–115
Ragusa PS, Bitterman A, Auerbach B, Healy WA 3rd (2016) Effectiveness of surgical safety checklists in improving patient safety. Orthopedics 39(2):e307–e310
Ramsay G, Haynes AB, Lipsitz SR, Solsky I, Leitch J, Gawande AA, Kumar M (2019) Reducing surgical mortality in Scotland by use of the WHO Surgical Safety Checklist. Br J Surg 106(8):1005–1011
Remiszewski DP, Bidra AS (2019) Implementation of a surgical safety checklist for dental implant surgeries in a prosthodontics residency program. J Prosthet Dent 122(4):371–375
Russ S, Rout S, Caris J, Mansell J, Davies R, Mayer E, Moorthy K, Darzi A, Vincent C, Sevdalis N (2015) Measuring variation in use of the WHO surgical safety checklist in the operating room: a multicenter prospective cross-sectional study. J Am Coll Surg 220:1–11
Russ S, Rout S, Sevdalis N, Moorthy K, Darzi A, Vincent C (2013) Do safety checklists improve teamwork and communication in the operating room? A systematic review. Ann Surg 258:856–871
Santana HT, Rodrigues MC, do Socorro Nantua Evangelista M (2016) Surgical teams' attitudes and opinions towards the safety of surgical procedures in public hospitals in the Brazilian federal district. BMC Res Notes 9:276
Schwendimann R, Milne J, Frush K, Ausserhofer D, Frankel A, Sexton JB (2013) A closer look at associations between hospital leadership walkrounds and patient safety climate and risk reduction: a cross-sectional study. Am J Med Qual 28(5):414–421
Seiden SC, Barach P (2006) Wrong-side/wrong-site, wrong-procedure, and wrong-patient adverse events: are they preventable? Arch Surg 141:931–939
Sewell M, Adebibe M, Jayakumar P, Jowett C, Kong K, Vemulapalli K, Levack B (2011) Use of the WHO surgical safety checklist in trauma and orthopedic patients. Int Orthop 35:897–901
Siddiqi A, Forte SA, Docter S, Bryant D, Sheth NP, Chen AF (2019) Perioperative antibiotic prophylaxis in total joint arthroplasty: a systematic review and meta-analysis. J Bone Joint Surg Am 101(9):828–842
Sobhy S, Zamora J, Dharmarajah K, Arroyo-Manzano D, Wilson M, Navaratnarajah R, Coomarasamy A, Khan KS, Thangaratinam S (2016) Anaesthesia-related maternal mortality in low-income and middle-income countries: a systematic review and meta-analysis. Lancet Glob Health 4(5):e320–e327
Sucupira E, Matta R, Zuker P, Matta J, Arbeláez JP, Uebel CO (2016) Aesthetic plastic surgery checklist: a safety tool. Aesthet Plast Surg 40(5):785–791
Takala RS, Pauniaho SL, Kotkansalo A, Helmiö P, Blomgren K, Helminen M, Kinnunen M, Takala A, Aaltonen R, Katila AJ, Peltomaa K, Ikonen TS (2011) A pilot study of the implementation of WHO surgical checklist in Finland: improvements in activities and communication. Acta Anaesthesiol Scand 55:1206–1214
Thomas EJ, Sexton JB, Neilands TB, Frankel A, Helmreich RL (2005) The effect of executive walk rounds on nurse safety climate attitudes: a randomized trial of clinical units. BMC Health Serv Res 5:28
Vats A, Vincent CA, Nagpal K, Davies RW, Darzi A, Moorthy K (2010) Practical challenges of introducing WHO surgical checklist: UK pilot experience. BMJ 340:54–63
Vila PM, Zenga J, Jackson RS (2017) Antibiotic prophylaxis in clean-contaminated head and neck surgery: a systematic review and meta-analysis. Otolaryngol Head Neck Surg 157(4):580–588
Vincent C, Moorthy K, Sarker SK, Chang A, Darzi AW (2004) Systems approaches to surgical quality and safety: from concept to measurement. Ann Surg 239 (4):475–482
Vivekanantham S, Ravindran RP, Shanmugarajah K, Maruthappu M, Shalhoub J (2014) Surgical safety checklists in developing countries. Int J Surg 12:2–6
Wang H, Zheng T, Chen D, Niu Z, Zhou X, Li S, Zhou Y, Cao S (2019) Impacts of the surgical safety checklist on postoperative clinical outcomes in gastrointestinal tumor patients: a single-center cohort study. Medicine (Baltimore) 98(28):e16418
Warnock G (2010) Of surgeons and safety checklists. Can J Surg 53(6):364–365
Wæhle HV, Harthug S, Søfteland E, Sevdalis N, Smith I, Wiig S, Aase K, Haugen AS (2019) Investigation of perioperative work processes in provision of antibiotic prophylaxis: a prospective descriptive qualitative study across surgical specialties in Norway. BMJ Open 9(6): e029671
W-Dahl A, Robertsson O, Stefánsdóttir A, Gustafson P, Lidgren L (2011) Timing of preoperative antibiotics for knee arthroplasties: improving the routines in Sweden. Patient Saf Surg 5:22
Weaver SJ, Lubomksi LH, Wilson RF, Pfoh ER, Martinez KA, Dy SM (2013) Promoting a culture of safety as a patient safety strategy. Ann Intern Med 158:369–374
Weiser TG, Regenbogen SE, Thompson KD, Haynes AB, Lipsitz SR, Berry WR, Gawande AA (2008) An estimation of the global volume of surgery: a modeling strategy based on available data. Lancet 372 (9633):139–144
WHO (2008a) Safe surgery saves lives. http://www.who.int/features/factfiles/safe_surgery/en/index.html. Accessed on 30 Nov 2020
WHO (2008b) Surgical safety checklist. https://www.who.int/patientsafety/safesurgery/tools_resources/SSSL_Checklist_finalJun08.pdf. Accessed on 30 Nov 2020
WHO (2009) Guidelines for safe surgery: safe surgery saves lives. https://apps.who.int/iris/bitstream/handle/10665/44185/9789241598552_eng.pdf?sequence=1&isAllowed=y. Accessed on 30 Nov 2020
Zavalkoff SR, Razack SI, Lavoie J, Dancea AB (2011) Handover after pediatric heart surgery: a simple tool improves information exchange. Pediatr Crit Care Med 12:309–313

Adv Exp Med Biol - Clinical and Experimental Biomedicine (2022) 13: 63–78
https://doi.org/10.1007/5584_2020_611

Published online: 31 December 2020

Benefit of Biological Drugs for Quality of Life in Patients with Ankylosing Spondylitis: A Systematic Review and Meta-Analysis of Clinical Trials

Wojciech Tański, Natalia Świątoniowska-Lonc, Krzysztof Dudek, and Beata Jankowska-Polańska

Abstract

Ankylosing spondylitis (AS) is a chronic inflammatory rheumatic disease involving the axial skeleton, peripheral joints, and extra-articular manifestations like psoriasis, inflammatory bowel disease, or uveitis. A deterioration of quality of life (QoL) affects the disease management and therapeutic decision-making. This meta-analysis focused on the influence of biological drugs on the QoL in SA compared to the effects of other therapeutic modalities. We searched the databases of MedLine, Academic Search Ultimate, CINAHL Complete, and Health Source – Nursing/Academic Edition for articles related to AS treatment using the terms "ankylosing spondylitis" OR "rheumatoid spondylitis" OR "spondylitis" AND "quality of life" OR "patient-reported outcomes" OR "well-being" OR "health-related quality of life" OR "biological treatment". The search came up with 10 English-language articles published between 2010 and 2020. Patients were evaluated with the following indexes and questionnaires: Assessment of Spondyloarthritis International Society (ASAS), Bath Ankylosing Spondylitis Disease Activity Index (BASDAI), Ankylosing Spondylitis Quality of Life (ASQoL), 36-Item Short-Form Health Survey (SF-36), Functional Assessment of Chronic Illness Therapy-Fatigue (FACIT-F), and the Bath Ankylosing Spondylitis Functional Index (BASFI), and Bath Ankylosing Spondylitis Functional (BASFI) Indexes. We found that the QoL, assessed with the ASQoL, improved significantly better in patients treated with biological drugs when compared to those treated with other standard therapies or placebo at a 4-month follow-up. However, improvements in other disease characteristics could not be differentiated based on the therapy modality. The finding that biological drugs are superior in improving the QoL should strengthen the recommendations for their use in patients with AS.

W. Tański
Department of Internal Medicine, Fourth Military Teaching Hospital, Wroclaw, Poland
e-mail: wtanski@op.pl

N. Świątoniowska-Lonc
Department of Clinical Nursing, Faculty of Health Science, Wroclaw Medical University, Wroclaw, Poland
e-mail: natalia.swiat@o2.pl

K. Dudek
Department of Transport Systems, Faculty of Mechanical Engineering, Wroclaw University of Technology, Wrocław, Poland
e-mail: krzysztof.dudek@pwr.edu.pl

B. Jankowska-Polańska (✉)
Department of Clinical Nursing, Faculty of Health Science, Wroclaw Medical University, Wroclaw, Poland
e-mail: beata.jankowska-polanska@umed.wroc.pl

Keywords

Ankylosing spondylitis · Biologic drugs · Disability · Inflammation · Patient management · Quality of life · Rheumatic disease · Rheumatic disease · Therapy

1 Introduction

Ankylosing spondylitis (AS) is a chronic inflammatory disorder characterized by a broad spectrum of clinical manifestations, laboratory abnormalities, and imaging features. The prevalence of AS in the general population is between 0.1% and 6%. The disease affects young people, and its incidence is highest in people in their thirties. The AS is associated with the presence of the HLA-B27 antigen, found in 90–95% of patients (Zhu et al. 2019). The underlying mechanisms are related to inflammatory, infectious, immunological, and genetic disorders. Typical symptoms include pain in the spine, chest, and peripheral joints, fatigue, stiffness, physical disability, fever, weight loss, and shortness of breath. The symptoms are hardly specific, which leads to delayed diagnosis and treatment. The AS may also involve non-articular tissues, notably the heart, lungs, eyes, or digestive tract, increasing the risk of premature death (Reveille and Weisman 2013).

AS treatment is based on non-steroidal anti-inflammatory drugs (NSAIDs). When these drugs are ineffective and high disease activity persists, clinically demonstrated by the Bath Ankylosing Spondylitis Disease Activity Index (BASDAI) score > 4 and the elevated erythrocyte sedimentation rate (ESR) and plasma C-reactive protein (CRP), biological drugs can be used. They offer considerable hope for effective treatment. Particularly, tumor necrosis factor-alpha (TNF-α) inhibitors appear effective. The introduction of biologicals in AS treatment has enabled the effective containment of the inflammatory process in patients with highly active and aggressive disease (Gao et al. 2012).

Rheumatic diseases are associated with an increased risk of organ pathology but also with a progressive disability and increased psychological burden. AS symptoms affect all aspects of patients' daily life. This leads to disease progression and disability which compromises fitness to work, work quality, daily activities, and, generally, health-related quality of life (QoL).

The interest in QoL dates to the 1970s and is associated with the holistic view of medicine. Therapeutic interventions are expected to prolong life and improve its quality. According to the positive concept of health, it is not the mere absence of disease but good physical and mental functioning and social adaptation. In clinical practice, QoL assessment complements objective indicators of outcome. It facilitates the selection of an optimal treatment protocol from the existing options. QoL assessment is based on patient self-reporting. It shows limitations in functioning, identifies areas where the patient experiences such limitations, and suggests priorities and preferences that may be relevant to further management planning (Megari 2013). In rheumatology, QoL has significant clinical implications but is not often addressed in practice. Studies are often limited to the assessment of correlations between basic symptoms of pain and stiffness and QoL. Concerning the impact of AS on QoL, studies show that patients suffer from impaired physical and mental health (Yang et al. 2016). However, few studies have yet addressed the influence of treatment with biological drugs on AS symptoms and QoL.

Rheumatologic patients usually associate the notion of health with functional status and quality of living with the disease. Management planning follows the alternating sequence of disease remission and exacerbation. The characteristics of rheumatic diseases make it difficult to establish long-term treatment objectives. When seeking the optimal treatment protocol, besides ways to delay the development of joint lesions and alleviate the associated symptoms, one must seek to improve the patient's daily functioning and his perceived QoL. To this end, QoL assessment should be an essential part of patient management and therapeutic decision-making. The purpose of this meta-analysis was to assess the QoL of patients with

AS, with the particular emphasis on the influence of using biological therapy on QoL as compared to the effects of other therapeutic modalities.

2 Methods

2.1 Search Strategies

This meta-analysis concerned the English-language articles published between 2010 and 2020 which addressed the features and therapy of AS. We performed a systematic searched of electronic databases such as PubMed, MedLine, Academic Search Ultimate, AHFS Consumer Medication Information, Open Dissertations, CINAHL Complete Dentistry and Oral Sciences, GreenFILE, Health Source – Consumer Edition, Health Source: Nursing/Academic Edition, International Pharmaceutical Abstracts, and MasterFILE Premier using the terms "ankylosing spondylitis" OR "rheumatoid spondylitis" OR "spondylitis" AND "quality of life" OR "patient-reported outcomes" OR "well-being" OR "health-related quality of life" OR "biological treatment". The search followed the Cochrane guidelines and was consistent with the Preferred Reporting Items for Systematic Review and Meta-Analysis (PRISMA) statement. Inclusion criteria consisted of age ≥18 years (7 studies), meeting the modified New York standards for ankylosing spondylitis (4 studies) or standards for axial ankylosing spondylitis in the Assessment of Spondyloarthritis International Society (ASAS) (3 studies), the need for daily treatment with NSAIDs or NSAIDs intolerance (4 studies), score ≥4 in the Bath Ankylosing Spondylitis Disease Activity Index (BASDAI), pain score ≥4 on the numeric rating scale (NRS 0–10) (6 studies), and written informed consent (4 studies). Out of the several hundred articles identified, the search came up with 10 relevant studies, conducted in 15 countries on 5 continents. A detailed methodological flow diagram is presented in Fig. 1. Studies that contained incomplete data, case reports, reviews, lack of QoL assessment, and studies on children were excluded.

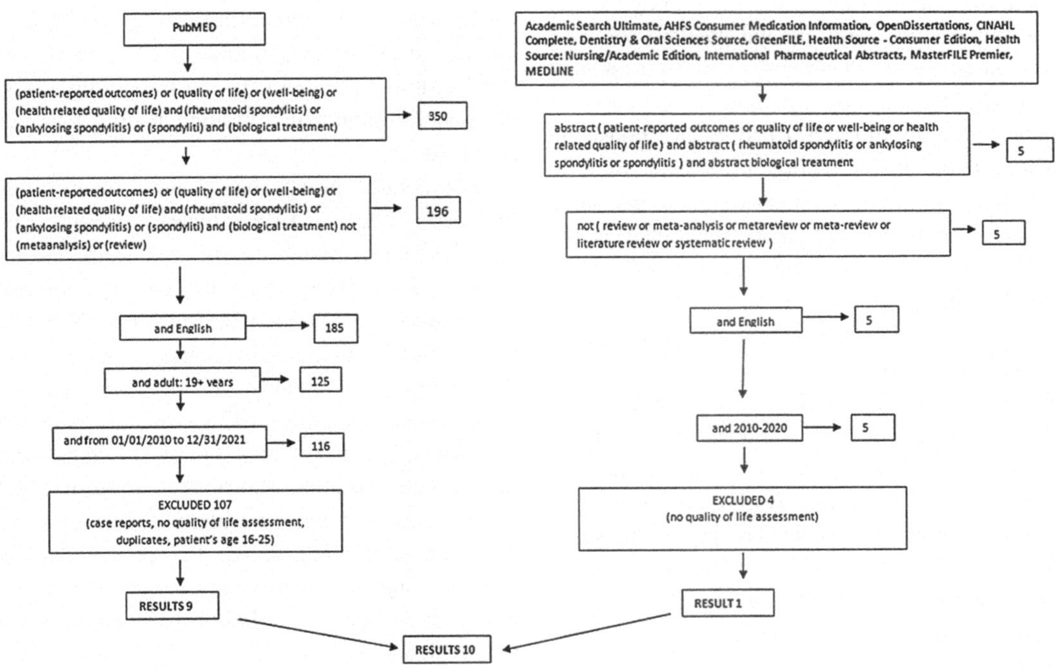

Fig. 1 Diagram showing the search-flow for the literature relevant for ankylosing spondylitis treatment

Questionnaire Structures The questionnaires used in the relevant studies were as follows: Bath Ankylosing Spondylitis Disease Activity Index (BASDAI), Ankylosing Spondylitis Quality of Life (ASQoL), 36-Item Short-Form Health Survey (SF-36), Functional Assessment of Chronic Illness Therapy-Fatigue (FACIT-F), and the Bath Ankylosing Spondylitis Functional Index (BASFI) (Rohde et al. 2020; van der Heijde et al. 2019; Fattahi et al. 2018a, b; Jafarnezhad-Ansariha et al. 2018; van der Heijde et al. 2018a, b; Arısoy et al. 2013; Pathan et al. 2013; Ertenli et al. 2012).

The ASQoL questionnaire is a disease-specific patient-reported outcome measure, based on the needs-model of QoL. It comprises 18 items, each with a dichotomous yes/no response option scored 1 and 0, respectively. A total score ranges from 0 to 18, with higher scores indicating a poorer QoL (Doward et al. 2003). The SF-36 is a 36-item questionnaire assessing the patient's health status. The questionnaire comprises eight domains: vitality, physical functioning, bodily pain, general health perception, physical role functioning, emotional role functioning, social role functioning, and mental health. Physical component score (PCS) and mental component score (MCS) may be calculated separately or along with eight domains of SF-36 Responses in each domain are converted to a scale of 0 to 100, with all items having assigned the same weight. The higher the score the better is the QoL (Ware Jr and Sherbourne 1992). The FACIT-F questionnaire covers four life domains of chronically ill patients. It comprises 5 parts: physical well-being (PWB) – 7 questions; social/family well-being (SWB) – 7 questions; emotional well-being (EWB) – 6 questions; functional well-being (FWB) – 7 questions, and fatigue subscale (FS) – 13 questions. Each question is rated on a five-point Likert scale. The higher the score the better is the QoL (Cella 1997). The BASFI questionnaire assesses the degree of functional limitation, with higher scores indicating a worse condition.

Literature articles were thoroughly screened by two reviewers for consistency with the subject of this meta-analysis above outlined. They determined if the content consists of interpretable patterns that sufficiently contribute to the accumulated knowledge and evidence-based practice and could advance the process of rehabilitation and care for SA patients. Any discrepancies in the reviewers' assessments were resolved by consensus. Data were extracted and put in the standardized forms that included general information, patient characteristics, study design, risk of bias according to the Newcastle-Ottawa Scale, and intermediate-to-long term (>6 months) main outcomes.

2.2 Study Groups

The active arm of this analysis included 593 patients (85.6% male) aged 22–60, suffering from AS for 1–21 years and treated with biological drugs. The main identified biological drugs used were the following: filgotinib (58 cases), adalimumab (92 cases), ixekizumab (164 cases), β-D-mannuronic acid (60 cases), apremilast (17 cases), infliximab (23 cases), and upadacitinib (89 cases). In the remaining cases, the generic nature of a biological drug was not provided.

The control group treated with other drugs included 702 (70.4% male) patients of 22–58 years of age, who suffered from AS for 1–18 years. They were treated by variable combinations of traditional drugs like NASIDs (582 cases), disease-modifying antirheumatic drugs (561) that notably included methotrexate (284 cases), analgesics (93 cases), and steroids (80 cases). In some studies, biological drugs were mixed with non-biological ones in an unstratified manner and were thus considered together. Aside from the used medications, 191 patients in the control group also received a placebo; 152 patients received a placebo in addition to other standard treatment and 39 patients received placebo alone.

2.3 Statistical Analysis

In this meta-analysis, we examined differences in the clinical improvements between SA patients treated with biological drugs (intervention group) and traditional non-biological drugs or placebo. In some studies, the drugs used were not stratified into types and thus were considered together. The effect-size (ES) was based on the standardized mean difference in a random or fixed model, based on the Q test of homogeneity. The random-effects model was used assuming that different studies would reflect different ES due to differences in patient samples and methods. In this model, the DerSimonian and Laird estimate with 95% confidence intervals (95%CI) were used, estimating the difference between the two groups based on the number of pooled standard deviations by which the two groups differed. This part of the analysis was performed using the R-software v3.6.2 for statistical computing for Windows. For the fixed model, Hedges' *g*, a bias-free measure of standardized mean differences, was used to estimate the ES, according to the formula: *g* x (mean-1 - mean-2)/SD*; where SD* is the pooled and weighted standard deviation of both study and control groups. The results were presented as forest plots. The total was calculated by assigning relative weights to treatment effects from the evaluated publications, depending on the sample size and standard error. A p-value of <0.05 defined a statistically significant difference. Calculations were performed using a commercial package of Statistica v13.3 software (StatSoft Inc; Tulsa, OK).

3 Results

3.1 Treatment of Ankylosing Spondylitis (AS)

The ASQoL assessment showed that patients treated with biological drugs showed a significantly better QoL at 4-month follow-up when compared to those treated with classical therapy alone (Hedges' *g* analysis for heterogeneity: df = 7, Q = 124.5, I^2 = 94.4%, $p < 0.001$, *vs.* df = 7, Q = 3.3, I^2 = 0.0%, p = 0.854, respectively), while both groups started from a similar baseline level of QoL (Fig. 2).

Since we found a beneficial influence on QoL of biological drugs in SA patients, we posed a question of whether the self-perceived improvement could relate to a particular biological drug used. The lack of standardization in studies on the effects of biological therapy makes it hard to compare patient outcomes. There are variably incomplete data, and different follow-up periods and instruments assessing the QoL and functional performance in the relevant studies surveyed. Nonetheless, we tallied the following information about the effects of single biological drugs.

Filgotinib – selective Janus kinase 1 (JAK1) inhibitor (*n* = *58*) (van der Heijde et al. 2018a) – treatment follow-up at 3 months. ASQoL score: baseline 12.8 ±3.5, follow-up 8.0 ±5.2 – improvement by 4.8 points; SF-36 PCS (physical): baseline 33.1 ±5.6, follow-up 41.6 ±7.9 – improvement by 8.5 points; SF-36 MCS (mental): baseline 43.7 ±11.1; follow-up 47.7 ±9.3 – improvement by 4.0 points.

Ixekizumab – monoclonal antibody against interleukin-17A, (van der Heijde et al. 2018b) – treatment follow-up at 4 months. Q2W (*n* = *83*): SF-36 PCS (physical): baseline 34.1 ±7.6, follow-up 42.1 ±0.8 – improvement by 8.0 points; Q4W (*n* = *81*): SF-36 MCS (mental): baseline 34.0 ±8.0, follow-up 41.7 ± 0.8 – improvement by 7.7 points.

β-D-mannuronic acid – marine algal polysaccharide (*n* = *30*) (Fattahi et al. 2018a, b; Jafarnezhad-Ansariha et al. 2018) – treatment follow-up at 3 months. ASQoL score: baseline 9.8 ±4.5; follow-up 6.6 ±4.6 – improvement by 3.2 points; baseline 9.1 ±0.7; follow-up 6.0 ±0.6 - improvement by 3.1 points; and baseline 9.8 ±4.5; follow-up 6.7 ±0.6 – improvement by 3.1 points, respectively.

Apremilast – phosphodiesterase 4 (PDE4) inhibitor (*n* = *17*) (Pathan et al. 2013) – treatment follow-up at 3 months. FACIT-F score:

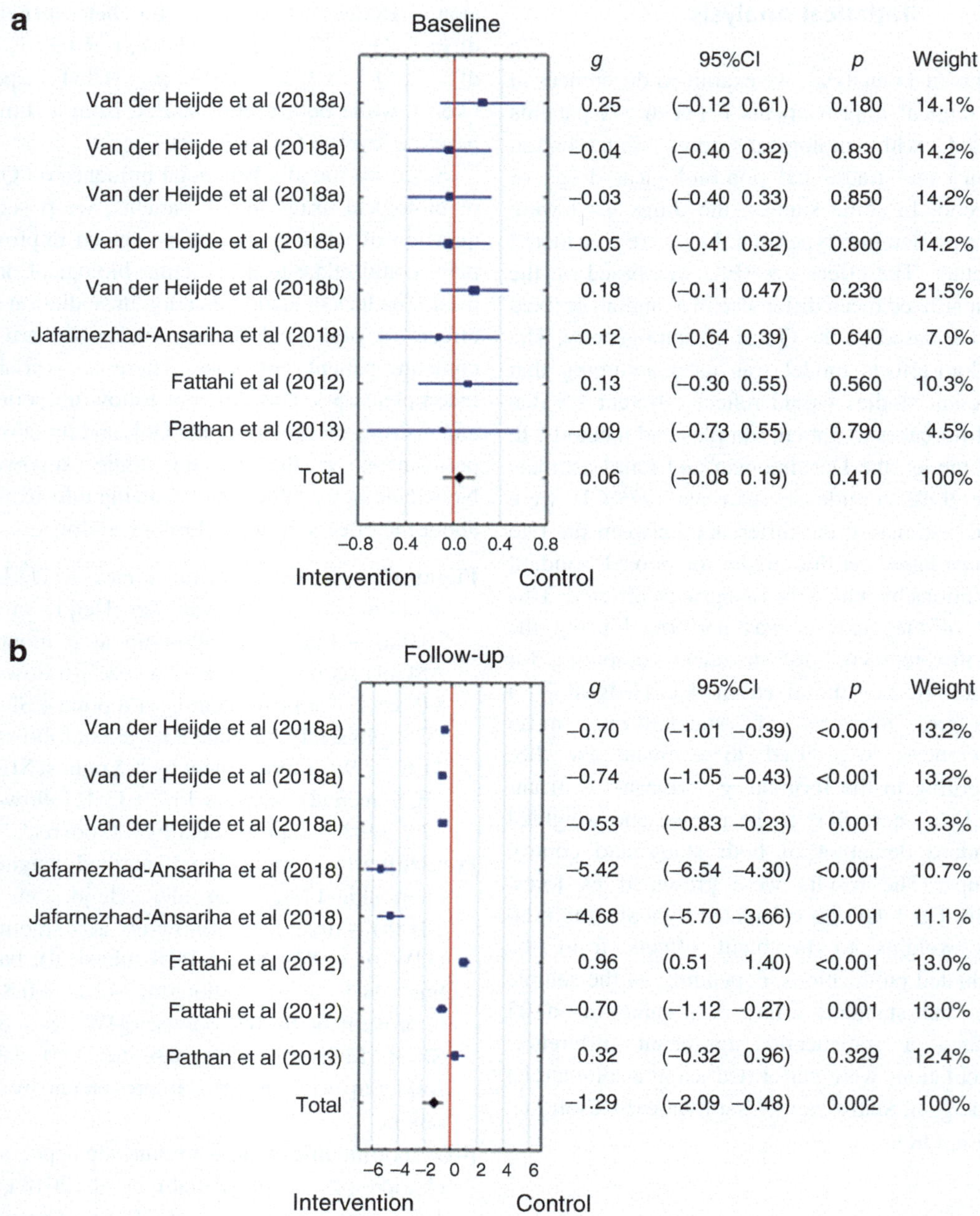

Fig. 2 Quality of life (QoL) in ankylosing spondylitis (AS) treated with biological drugs (intervention group) when compared to the control group not using biological drugs, assessed with ASQoL, except for a study of Pathan et al. (2013), where the FACIT-F questionnaire was used. Note no difference in QoL between the two groups at onset (**a**) and a distinctly better QoL at a 4-month follow-up (**b**)

baseline 107.8 ±25.7, follow-up 117.1 – improvement by 9.3 points. The improvement concerned the physical, social, and emotional domains, as well as the fatigue.

Upadacitinib – Janus kinase (JAK) inhibitor (Van der Heijde et al. 2019) – QoL improvement was verified based on the difference between the biological *versus* non-biological treatment due to the unspecified treatment follow-up period.

The superior quality of life, assessed with the ASQoL questionnaire, was the single parameter found in this meta-analysis with benefits related to the implementation of treatment with biological drugs. All the other measurements showed improvements in response to treatment, irrespective of biological or traditional drugs used, or even placebo. Therefore, in further analysis, all the drugs were grouped. The AS disease activity, assessed on the BADSI scale, improved from baseline to follow-up while using biologicals (Fig. 3). However, a positive trend of improving the functional performance was also observed with traditional treatments as well as placebo, regardless of the treatment duration (Table 1).

Besides disease activity level, C-reactive protein (CRP) in blood plasma, a marker of inflammation in AS patients, is relevant for the monitoring of treatment effects. Figure 4 shows a significant drop in CRP levels after treatment with biological drugs ($p = 0.001$ for the entire group; Hedges' *g* analysis). A decline in CRP was noted while using all individual biological drugs included in the analysis except for one case when its level tended to rise after treatment with β-D-mannuronic acid (Jafarnezhad-Ansariha et al. 2018). However, CRP also declined while using other drugs, with a single exception of placebo in a study by Van der Heijde et al. (2018a). Detailed results for biological and other drugs are displayed in Table 2.

In the management of AS patients, the American College of Rheumatology (ACR) recommends the comprehensive ASAS assessment of the

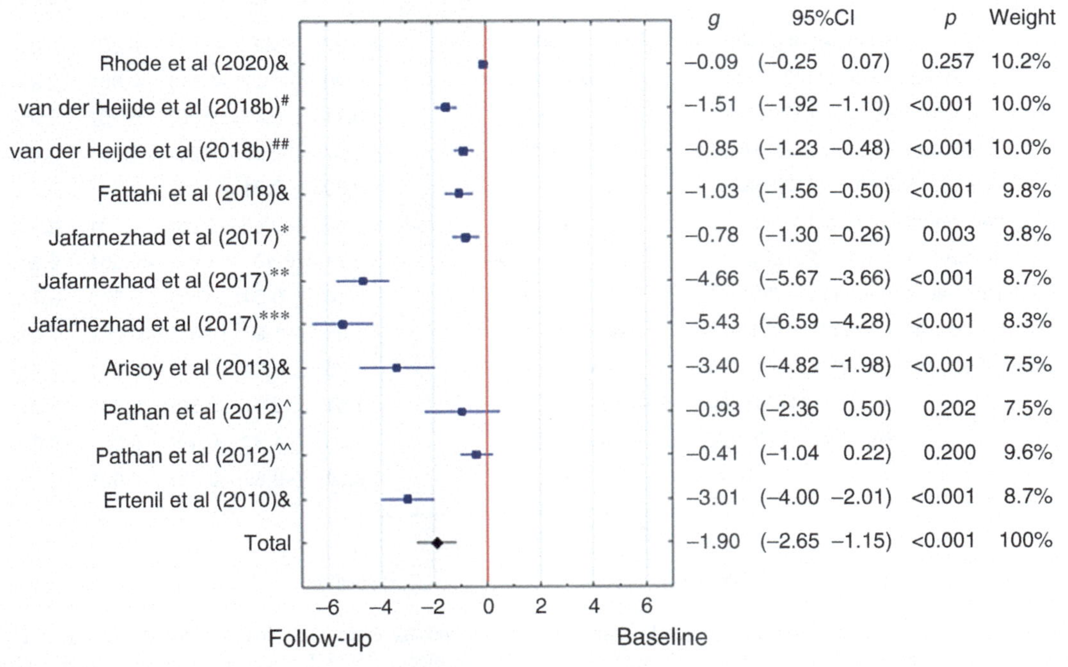

Fig. 3 Disease activity level in ankylosing spondylitis (AS) in patients treated with both biological and traditional drugs at baseline and follow-up after treatment, assessed with the Bath Ankylosing Spondylitis Disease Activity Index (BASDAI). The random-effects model with Hedges' *g*. The effect size and confidence interval for each study appear graphically on a separate row (blue). The summary effect and its confidence interval are displayed at the bottom (black). 95% CI, lower and upper 95% confidence intervals; [&]drugs unstratified, [#]filgotinib, [##]placebo, *β-D-mannuronic acid, **naproxen, ***placebo, ^apremilast, ^^placebo

Table 1 Disease activity level in ankylosing spondylitis (AS) in patients treated with both biological and traditional drugs at baseline and follow-up after treatment, assessed on the Bath Ankylosing Spondylitis Disease Activity Index (BASDAI) at baseline and follow-up after treatment, considering all drugs

Source	Treatment	Baseline		Follow-up		
		Patients (n)	Score	Months	Patients (n)	Score
Rohde et al. (2020)	Drugs unstratified	380	3.1 ±2.1	60	240	2.9 ±2.2
Van der Heijde et al. (2018a)	Filgotinib	58	6.9 ±1.2	3	58	4.5 ±2.0
	Placebo	58	7.0 ±1.3	3	58	5.6 ±1.9
Fattahi et al. (2018a)	Drugs unstratified	30	5.8 ±1.3	4	30	4.1 ±1.9
Jafarnezhad-Ansariha et al. (2018)	β-D-mannuronic acid	30	5.8 ±0.2	4	30	5.5 ±0.5
	Naproxen	28	5.7 ±0.2	4	28	3.9 ±0.5
	Placebo	27	5.9 ±0.2	4	27	3.8 ±0.5
Arısoy et al. (2013)	Drugs unstratified	9	7.0 ±1.1	4	9	2.1 ±1.6
Pathan et al. (2013)	Apremilast	17	4.8 ±2.2	4	17	3.2 ±1.6
	Placebo	19	4.4 ±1.8	4	19	3.6 ±2.0
Ertenli et al. (2012)	Drugs unstratified	16	6.0 ±1.2	4	16	2.3 ±1.2

Scores are means ±SD

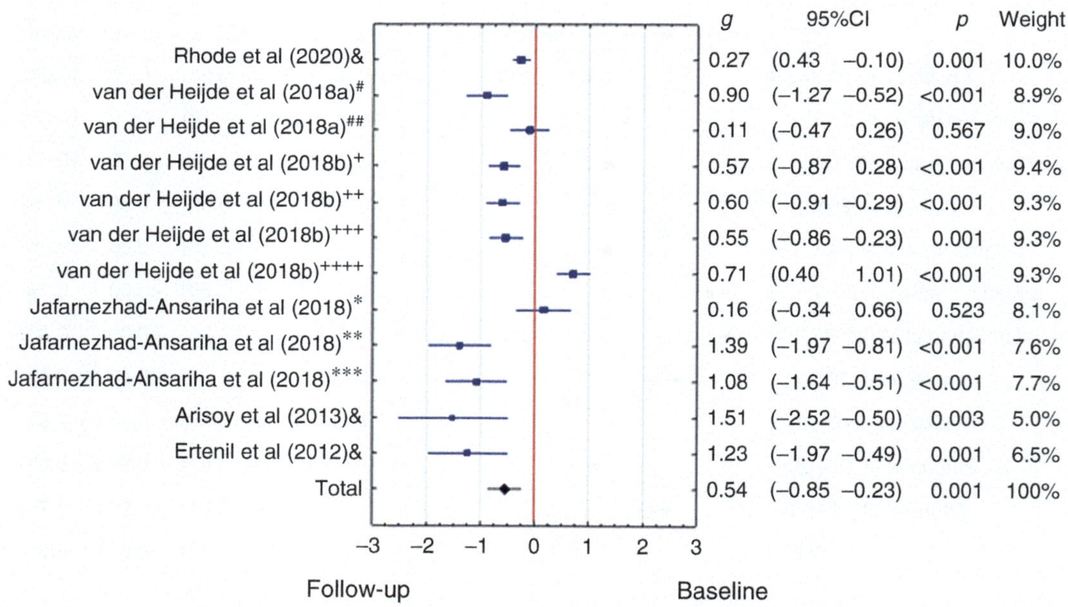

Fig. 4 C-reactive protein (CRP) in the blood plasma of ankylosing spondylitis (AS) patients treated with biological and traditional drugs at baseline and follow-up after treatment. The random-effects model with Hedges' *g*. The effect size and confidence interval for each study appear graphically on a separate row (blue). The summary effect and its confidence interval are displayed at the bottom (black). 95% CI, lower and upper 95% confidence intervals; &drugs unstratified, #filgotinib, ##placebo, +adalimumab, ++ixekizumab Q2W, +++ixekizumab Q4W, ++++placebo, *β-D-mannuronic acid, **naproxen, ***placebo

Table 2 C-reactive protein (CRP) in the blood plasma of ankylosing spondylitis (AS) patients at baseline and treatment follow-up, considering all drugs

Source	Treatment	Baseline		Follow-up		
		Patients (n)	mg/L	Months	Patients (n)	mg/L
Rohde et al. (2020)	Drugs unstratified	380	10.0 ±13.2	60	240	6.7 ±10.7
Van der Heijde et al. (2018b)	Filgotinib	58	19.6 ±13.3	3	58	8.8 ±10.5
	Placebo	58	21.2 ±23.0	3	58	18.9 ±20.2
Van der Heijde et al. (2018a)	Adalimumab	90	12.5 ±17.6	4	90	5.3 ±1.9
	Ixekizumab Q2W	83	13.4 ±15.3	4	83	6.8 ±2.0
	Ixekizumab Q4W	81	12.2 ±13.3	4	81	7.1 ±2.0
	Placebo	87	16.0 ±2.1	4	87	17.4 ±1.9
Jafarnezhad-Ansariha et al. (2018)	β-D-mannuronic acid	30	8.3 ±1.2	4	30	8.5 ±1.1
	Naproxen	28	8.0 ±0.8	4	28	6.8 ±0.9
	Placebo	27	8.1 ±0.9	4	27	7.0 ±1.1
Arısoy et al. (2013)	Drugs unstratified	9	22.9 ±15.0	1.5	9	5.2 ±4.9
Ertenli et al. (2012)	Drugs unstratified	16	3.7 ±3.5	1.5	16	0.6 ±0.5

Scores are means ±SD

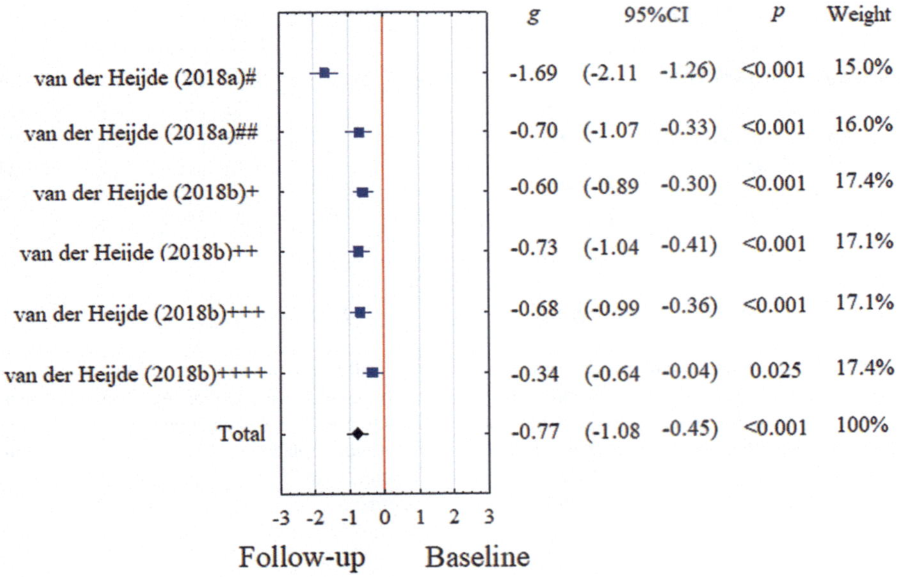

Fig. 5 Effectiveness of clinical treatment using biological drugs and placebo in ankylosing spondylitis (AS) patients, based on the SpondyloArthritis International Society (ASAS) assessment at baseline and follow-up after treatment. The random-effects model with Hedges' *g*. The effect size and confidence interval for each study appear graphically on a separate row (blue). The summary effect and its confidence interval are displayed at the bottom (black). 95% CI, lower and upper 95% confidence intervals; #filgotinib, ##placebo, +adalimumab, ++ixekizumab Q2W, +++ixekizumab Q4W, ++++placebo

patient's functioning, which is used as a criterion for initiating biological therapy (Ward et al. 2016). In our meta-analysis, a comparison of ASAS scores at baseline and follow-up after treatment showed a significant improvement in functioning in patients using biological drugs as well as in those receiving a placebo, with inappreciable differences (Fig. 5 and Table 3).

Table 3 SpondyloArthritis International Society (ASAS) scoring in ankylosing spondylitis (AS) patients at baseline and treatment follow-up, considering biological drugs and placebo

Source	Treatment	Baseline		Follow-up		
		Patients (n)	Score	(Months)	Patients (n)	Score
Van der Heijde et al. (2018b)	Filgotinib	58	4.2 ±0.6	3	58	2.8 ±1.0
	Placebo	58	4.2 ±0.8	3	58	3.6 ±0.9
Van der Heijde et al. (2018a)	Adalimumab	90	8.2 ±3.7	4	90	5.9 ±4.0
	Ixekizumab Q2W	83	8.4 ±3.6	4	83	5.7 ±3.9
	Ixekizumab Q4W	81	7.5 ±3.3	4	81	5.1 ±3.6
	Placebo	87	8.1 ±3.5	4	87	6.9 ±3.8

Scores are means ±SD

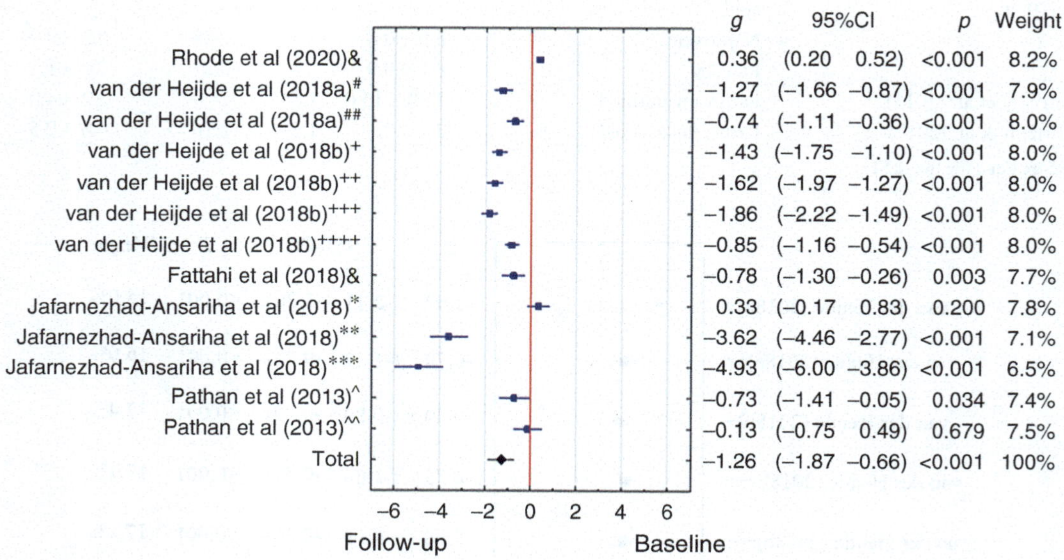

Fig. 6 Functional assessment in ankylosing spondylitis (AS) patients treated with biological and traditional drugs at baseline and treatment follow-up, based on the Bath Ankylosing Spondylitis Functional Index (BASFI) questionnaire. The random-effects model with Hedges' *g*. The effect size and confidence interval for each study appear graphically on a separate row (blue). The summary effect and its confidence interval are displayed at the bottom (black). 95% CI, lower and upper 95% confidence intervals; *filgotinib, **placebo, +adalimumab, ++ixekizumab Q2W, +++ixekizumab Q4W, ++++placebo, #β-D-mannuronic acid, ##naproxen, ###placebo, ^apremilast, ^^placebo

The evaluation of functional performance in the AS patients using the BASFI also showed, overall, significant score decreases pointing to improvements, irrespective of the therapy mode (Fig. 6). There were, however, single exceptions to the opposite. Rohde et al. (2020) noticed no improvement in the BASFI score (2.6 *vs.* 3.4; p >0.05) in a group of patients treated with biological drugs at a 5-year follow-up. Likewise, no functional improvement was noticed while using a placebo (4.7 *vs.* 5.8; p >0.05) in a study of Jafarnezhad-Ansariha et al. (2018) (Table 4).

Table 4 Functional assessment in AS patients based on the Bath Ankylosing Spondylitis Functional Index (BASFI) at baseline and follow-up after treatment, considering all drugs

		Baseline		Follow-up		
Study	Treatment	Patients (n)	Score	Months	Patients (n)	Score
Rohde et al. (2020)	Drugs unstratified	380	2.6 ±2.2	60	240	3.4 ±2.2
Van der Heijde et al. (2018a)	Filgotinib	58	7.0 ±1.5	3	58	4. 6 ±2.2
	Placebo	58	6.9 ±1.6	3	58	5.6 ±1.9
Van der Heijde et al. (2018b)	Adalimumab	90	6.1 ±2.1	4	90	4.0 ±0.2
	Ixekizumab Q2W	83	6.3 ±2.1	4	83	3.9 ±0.2
	Ixekizumab Q4W	81	6.1 ±1.8	4	81	3.7 ±0.2
	Placebo	87	6.4 ±1.9	4	87	5.2 ±0.2
Fattahi et al. (2018a)	Drugs unstratified	30	4.4 ±2.0	3	30	2.9 ±1.8
Jafarnezhad-Ansariha et al. (2018)	β-D-mannuronic acid	30	4.4 ±0.3	3	30	3.3 ±0.3
	Naproxen	28	4.2 ±0.3	3	28	2.7 ±0.3
	Placebo	27	4.7 ±0.3	3	27	5.8 ±0.3
Pathan et al. (2013)	Apremilast	17	4.6 ±2.4	3	17	2.8 ±2.2
	Placebo	19	3.5 ±2.2	3	19	3.2 ±2.0

Scores are means ±SD

Table 5 Factors affecting the quality of life (QoL) in ankylosing spondylitis (AS) patients

Factors increasing QoL	Factors decreasing QoL
Younger age, higher education, lower disease burden, low BASDAI, high BAS-G, high CRP, no use of biological treatment at baseline, and low HAQ score (Rohde et al. 2020), upadactinib 15 mg once a day (van der Heijde et al. 2019), filgotinib (van der Heijde et al. 2018a), adalimumab and ixekizumab (van der Heijde et al. 2018b), β-D-mannuronic acid, naproxen, lower CRP, and longer time elapsing from the intervention (Arısoy et al. 2013), apremilast (Pathan et al. 2013)	Anxiety and depression, erythrocyte sedimentation rate, Bath Ankylosing Spondylitis Disease Activity Index (BASDAI) score (Arısoy et al. 2013)

3.2 Positive and Negative Predictors of Quality of Life (QoL) in Patients with Ankylosing Spondylitis (AS)

Besides QoL scoring, the research on QoL often includes the search for the presaged predictors of QoL. In the relevant publications, the following factors are listed as positive predictors: age, social support, professional activity, illness acceptance, and rehabilitation. Conversely, negative predictors are the following: living alone, depression, severe symptoms, pain, frequent hospitalizations, and old age (Jankowska-Polanska et al. 2017; Polanski et al. 2016). The present meta-analysis revealed that positive predictors for QoL among patients with AS included younger age, better education, lower symptom severity, treatment with biologicals and other selected drugs, and shorter treatment duration. The adverse predictors were anxiety and depression, and greater symptom severity. These results are summarized in Table 5.

Biological drugs are recommended for SA patients who do not respond to other drugs over 6 months' treatment. These drugs, however, have adverse events that are displayed and compared against placebo in Fig. 7. The most often in decreasing frequency are the following: infections, inclusive of upper respiratory tract infections (133 patients), neutropenia grade 1 (32 patients), headache (31 patients), and injection site reactions (25 patients). Out of these

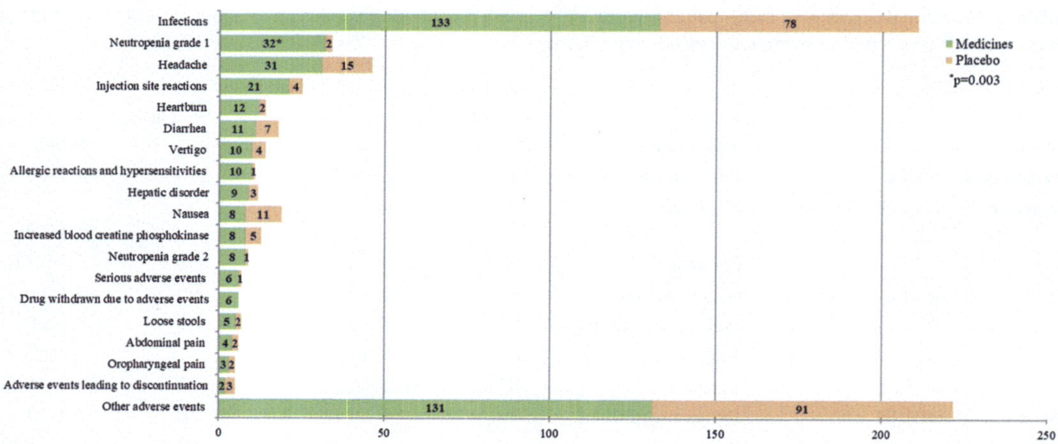

Fig. 7 Adverse effects in ankylosing spondylitis (AS) patients treated with biological drugs *versus* placebo; *significant difference between biological drugs and placebo

events, neutropenia grade 1 occurred significantly more often in patients treated with biological drugs (adaliumumab Q2W, ixekizumab Q2W, and ixekizumab Q4W) than placebo; 5.7% versus 0.6%, respectively ($p = 0.003$). The incidence of the other treatment-associated adverse events differed insignificantly between the biological drugs and placebo.

4 Discussion

According to the New York criteria, AS affects 0.007–1.7% of the global population, with an annual incidence of 0.44–7.3 *per* 100,000 individuals (Stolwijk et al. 2012). The prevalence in central Europe is estimated at 0.5% and most patients are men. It is a potentially serious disease with a variety of symptoms, typically requiring multidisciplinary treatment coordinated by a rheumatologist. Treatment for AS is complex, comprising medicines, physiotherapy, psychotherapy, and surgical interventions. The severity of chronic pain and stiffness increases gradually as the inflammation spreads to higher segments of the spine, disrupting its normal curvature. The associated ankylosis, peripheral joint deformities, and extremity contractures often lead to severe disability. As the disease often affects young people, most commonly in their thirties, it interferes with professional and social activity. About 10–30% of patients give up professional activity within 10 years of disease onset due to the progressive functional restriction. The available literature indicates that the life expectancy of AS patients is shorter than that in the general population due to disease complications (Haroon et al. 2015). This meta-analysis shows that biological drugs used in SA offer the benefit of a better patient QoL compared with the traditional non-biological treatment. Both kinds of treatments have the potential to generate a similar specter of multi-system adverse effects during a long-term follow-up. Biological drugs, noticeably, significantly more often may cause mild neutropenia than do non-biological ones. Nonetheless, the advantage of QoL with biological drugs provides a rationale to consider them as the more effective option.

The main objective of AS treatment is achieving the best possible QoL in the long term, by managing symptoms and inflammation, preventing progressive structural damage, and maintaining or restoring functional performance and ability to participate in social activities. For more than 10 years, biological drugs have been used as a pharmacological tool for AS treatment in Poland, with a lot of hope placed in these medications by physicians and patients alike. The drugs in use are monoclonal antibodies that bind to humoral factors and cells involved in the immune response, thus inhibiting inflammation. Their application provides benefits like a rapid effect, symptom alleviation, longer periods of remission, a lower level of pain, and better QoL. Notably, QoL in terms of physical functioning is enhanced more than that of mental health (Law et al. 2018). Gorman et al. (2002) have reported that etanercept produces significant improvements in morning stiffness, spinal pain, number of swollen joints, and functional performance in AS patients. Studies on the use of TNF-α inhibitors in AS treatment also show less pain and improvements in functional activity and performance and laboratory tests, including blood CRP levels (Tłustochowicz 2011). In this meta-analysis, we also found a downward trend in CRP blood content, taken as a clinical index of treatment effectiveness. Likewise, in a study performed at the Institute of Rheumatology in Prague, Chechia, nearly one-half of AS patients treated with biological drugs had a positive and effective clinical response (Lachaine et al. 2013). In a study by van der Heijde et al. (2018b), patients treated with adalimumab showed an improvement in QoL at a 3–6-month follow-up, sustained for 5 years despite the signs of inflammation found in X-ray images. The improvement was particularly clear while using the BASFI and ASQoL questionnaires. According to those authors, the QoL is mainly determined by functional performance and disease activity. On the other side, the physical domain of QoL is affected by spine mobility and disease activity determined by the irreversible structural damage and reversible inflammation in the spine (Machado et al. 2010). Rohde et al. (2020) have found that patients with axial spondyloarthritis do not show a deterioration in health-related QoL during 5 years of treatment with biological drugs but have a significant improvement in physical health evaluated by the generic SF-36 questionnaire. In another study, the administration of 15 mg of upadacitimid once daily produced a response 2 weeks after treatment onset in SA patients, consisting of back pain reduction that lasted for 14 consecutive weeks and was confirmed by abating inflammation of the spine and sacroiliac joints in the magnetic resonance imaging (van der Heijde et al. 2019). The authors have documented that improvements in functioning and a reduction in disease activity were greater in patients treated with biological drugs than in those receiving placebo, with adverse events being of no major concern or requiring a change or discontinuation of therapy. However, patients treated with the biological drug had a higher creatinine kinase level, albeit not associated with more severe functional impairment.

In another study, the effect of filgotinib was assessed, with the primary endpoint being a change in disease activity from the baseline level (van der Heijde et al. 2018a). At a 3-month follow-up, the mean ankylosing spondylitis disease activity score (ASDAS) was higher in the filgotinib group when compared to placebo, showing the effectiveness of the drug in reducing symptoms of AS inflammation. The biological drug was well tolerated. The incidence of adverse events in the biological therapy group was akin to that in the placebo group as also was the number of patients who discontinued the treatment. In a different study by van der Heijde et al. (2018b), ixekizumab was administered every 3 or 4 weeks and its effects were compared against placebo. At a 4-month follow-up, physical function improved, and the disease activity was lower in patients treated with the biological drug, and the improvements were greater than those possibly observed with placebo. No difference was found concerning adverse events between the biological drug and placebo.

Another biological drug, proven effective in SA, is β-D-mannuronic acid (Fattahi et al. 2018a). The drug appeared effective 2 weeks after treatment onset and over 3 months of continued therapy. Likewise, improvements mainly concerned the disease activity and functional performance. This study did not compare the drug with a placebo. In another study, Jafarnezhad-Ansariha et al. (2018) have compared the therapeutic effectiveness of β-D-mannuronic acid to a combination of naproxen and placebo. The outcome measure was a mean change from baseline to therapy week 12. The authors show beneficial effects of the drug in that it reduced pain, stiffness, and inflammation assessed by the blood CRP level, as well as improvements in physical function assessed by BASDAI and BASFI scores. Further, treatment-associated adverse events did not exceed those observed in the control treatment consisting of naproxen and placebo. Fattahi et al. (2018b) have also compared the therapeutic effectiveness of β-D-mannuronic against naproxen with placebo and confirmed good tolerance and high effectiveness of the biological drug over a 3-month follow-up. Beneficial effects included less pain, better functional performance, and lower CRP levels. In this study, the biological drug was associated with fewer adverse events compared to naproxen. On the other hand, Pathan et al. (2013) have investigated the treatment with an oral phosphodiesterase 4 inhibitor, apremilast, on the premise that it might be effective and well-tolerated in AS patients as it modulates biomarkers of bone biology. The study, however, has failed to establish the presence of appreciable benefits at a 3-month follow-up compared to placebo.

The known effects of biological drugs are not limited to the inhibition of disease progression, improvements in functional status, and reductions in stiffness, pain, and inflammation. Studies have shown the effectiveness of TNF-α inhibitors, e.g., infliximab, in the treatment of depressive symptoms accompanying the AS (Arısoy et al. 2013). In a study by Ertenli et al. (2012), infusions of infliximab were associated with a gradual reduction of depression and anxiety symptoms and QoL improvements since the very beginning of the intervention, and the drug's effectiveness increased with consecutive infusions.

Among predictors of QoL, the literature notably mentions higher education associating with a better long-term health-related QoL (Kotsis et al. 2014). The relation of patient age to the QoL remains somehow debatable. A younger age often means a shorter duration of illness, and thus, less structural damage and fewer complications (Rohde et al. 2020). On the other hand, the duration of illness is difficult to establish in patients with axial SA as symptoms may develop for up to 10 years before the diagnosis is made (Feldtkeller et al. 2000).

A major limitation of this meta-analysis is a lack of standardized data in all papers included in it, which concerns the research instruments used, intervention duration, and inclusion or not of a control group. Moreover, the scoring of instruments is not always compatible with each other in different papers, which hampers the interpretation of findings. Another limitation is the use of different active substances and different follow-up periods across the studies. Additionally, some studies included the assessment at just two-time points whereas repeated assessments at multiple equal intervals would have produced clearer results.

5 Conclusions

We conclude that patients suffering from ankylosing spondylitis, generally, benefit from regular treatment concerning QoL and functional performance. The benefits are greater with biological therapy than with using a placebo. The QoL is positively influenced by younger age, higher education, better functional status, biological therapy, and a longer of treatment, and negatively influenced by anxiety and depression. There appears no appreciable difference concerning the adverse events between biological and standard therapy, except for the propensity for neutropenia that is more common in the biologically treated patients. To achieve a well-scrutinized view on ankylosing spondylitis treatment, it is recommendable that future evaluations be based on studies that involve the controlled use of the same drug and employ the same standardized research instruments. Nonetheless, we believe that the finding that biological drugs are superior in improving the QoL should strengthen the recommendations for their use in patients with AS.

Conflicts of Interest The authors declare no conflicts of interest in relation to this article.

Ethical Approval This review article does not contain any studies with human participants or animals performed by any of the authors.

References

Arısoy O, Bes C, Cifci C, Sercan M, Soy M (2013) The effect of TNF-alpha blockers on psychometric measures in ankylosing spondylitis patients: a preliminary observation. Rheumatol Int 33:1855–1864

Cella D (1997) Manual of the Functional Assessment of Chronic Illness Therapy (FACIT) Measurement System. Center on Outcomes, Research and Education (CORE). Version 4. Evanston Northwestern Healthcare and Northwestern University, Evanston, IL

Doward LC, Spoorenberg A, Cook AS, Whalley D, Helliwell PS, Kay LJ, McKenna SP, Tennant A, van der Heijde D, Chamberlain MA (2003) Development of the ASQoL: a quality of life instrument specific to ankylosing spondylitis. Ann Rheum Dis 62(1):20–26

Ertenli I, Ozer S, Kiraz S, Apras SB, Akdogan A, Karadag O, Calguneri M, Kalyoncu U (2012) Infliximab, a TNF-alpha antagonist treatment in patients with ankylosing spondylitis: the impact on depression, anxiety and quality of life level. Rheumatol Int 32(2):323–330

Fattahi MJ, Ahmadi H, Jafarnezhad-Ansariha F, Mortazavi-Jahromi SS, Rehm BHA, Cuzzocrea S, Matsuo H, Mirshafiey A (2018a) Oral administration effects of β-d-mannuronic acid (M2000) on Th17 and regulatory T cells in patients with ankylosing spondylitis. Biomed Pharmacother 100:495–500

Fattahi MJ, Jamshidi AR, Mahmoudi M, Vojdanian M, Yekaninejad MS, Jafarnezhad-Ansariha F, Ahmadi H, Rehm BHA, Matsuo H, Cuzzocrea S, Hosseini M, Hashemi SN, Aghazadeh Z, Mirshafiey A (2018b) Evaluation of the efficacy and safety of β-D-mannuronic acid in patients with ankylosing spondylitis: a 12-week randomized, placebo-controlled, phase I/II clinical trial. Int Immunopharmacol 54:112–117

Feldtkeller E, Bruckel J, Khan MA (2000) Scientific contributions of ankylosing spondylitis patient advocacy groups. Curr Opin Rheumatol 12(4):239–247

Gao X, Wendling D, Botteman MF, Carter JA, Rao S, Cifaldi M (2012) Clinical and economic burden of extra-articular manifestations in ankylosing spondylitis patients treated with anti-tumor necrosis factor agents. J Med Econ 15(6):1054–1063

Gorman JD, Sack KE, Davis JC Jr (2002) Treatment of ankylosing spondylitis by inhibition of tumor necrosis factor alpha. N Engl J Med 346(18):1349–1356

Haroon NN, Paterson JM, Li P, Inman RD, Haroon N (2015) Patients with ankylosing spondylitis have increased cardiovascular and cerebrovascular mortality: a population-based study. Ann Intern Med 163 (6):409–416

Jafarnezhad-Ansariha F, Yekaninejad MS, Jamshidi A, Mansouri R, Vojdanian M, Mahmoudi M, Fattahi MJ, Hashemi SN, Rehm BHA, Matsuo H, Esposito E, Cuzzocrea S, Mirshafiey A (2018) The effects of β-D-mannuronic acid (M2000), as a novel NASID, on COX1 and COX2 activities and gene expression in ankylosing spondylitis patients and the murine monocyte/macrophage, J774 cell line. Inflammopharmacology 26(2):375–384

Jankowska-Polanska B, Uchmanowicz I, Wysocka A, Uchmanowicz B, Lomper K, Fal AM (2017) Factors affecting the quality of life of chronic dialysis patients. Eur J Pub Health 27(2):262–267

Kotsis K, Voulgari PV, Drosos AA, Carvalho AF, Hyphantis T (2014) Health-related quality of life in patients with ankylosing spondylitis: a comprehensive review. Expert Rev Pharmacoecon Outcomes Res 14 (6):857–872

Lachaine J, Beauchemin C, Desjardins O (2013) Use of biological agents in the treatment of rheumatoid arthritis: an analysis of the Quebec provincial drug reimbursement program database. Value Health 3:230–231

Law L, Rehnman JB, Deminger A, Klingberg E, Jacobsson LTH, Forsblad-d'Elia H (2018) Factors related to health-related quality of life in ankylosing spondylitis, overall and stratified by sex. Arthritis Res Ther 20(1):284

Machado P, Landewé R, Braun J, Hermann KA, Baker D, van der Heijde D (2010) Both structural damage and inflammation of the spine contribute to impairment of spinal mobility in patients with ankylosing spondylitis. Ann Rheum Dis 69(8):1465–1470

Megari K (2013) Quality of life in chronic disease patients. Health Psychol Res 1(3):e27

Pathan E, Abraham S, Van Rossen E, Withrington R, Keat A, Charles PJ, Paterson E, Chowdhury M, McClinton C, Taylor PC (2013) Efficacy and safety of apremilast, an oral phosphodiesterase 4 inhibitor, in ankylosing spondylitis. Ann Rheum Dis 72 (9):1475–1480

Polanski J, Jankowska-Polanska B, Rosinczuk J, Chabowski M, Szymanska-Chabowska A (2016) Quality of life of patients with lung cancer. Onco Targets Ther 9:1023–1028

Reveille JD, Weisman MH (2013) The epidemiology of back pain, axial spondyloarthritis and HLA-B27 in the United States. Am J Med Sci 345:431–436

Rohde G, Berg KH, Pripp AH, Prřven A, Haugeberg G (2020) No deterioration in health-related quality of life in patients with axial spondyloarthritis followed for 5 years in ordinary outpatient clinics in the biological treatment era. Qual Life Res 29:99–107

Stolwijk C, Boonen A, van Tubergen A, Reveille JD (2012) Epidemiology of spondyloarthritis. Rheum Dis Clin N Am 38(3):441–476

Tłustochowicz M (2011) Rytuksymab in treatment of rheumatoid arthritis. Reumatologia 49(1):55–61. (Article in Polish)

van der Heijde D, Baraliakos X, Gensler LS, Maksymowych WP, Tseluyko V, Nadashkevich O, Abi-Saab W, Tasset C, Meuleners L, Besuyen R, Hendrikx T, Mozaffarian N, Liu K, Greer JM, Deodhar A, Landewé R (2018a) Efficacy and safety of filgotinib, a selective Janus kinase 1 inhibitor, in patients with active ankylosing spondylitis (TORTUGA): results from a randomised, placebo-controlled, phase 2 trial. Lancet 392 (10162):2378–2387

van der Heijde D, Cheng-Chung Wei J, Dougados M, Mease P, Deodhar A, Maksymowych WP, Van den Bosch F, Sieper J, Tomita T, Landewé R, Zhao F, Krishnan E, Adams DH, Pangallo B, Carlier H, COAST-V study group (2018b) Ixekizumab, an interleukin-17A antagonist in the treatment of ankylosing spondylitis or radiographic axial spondyloarthritis in patients previously untreated with biological disease-modifying anti-rheumatic drugs (COAST-V): 16 week results of a phase 3 randomised, double-blind, active-controlled and placebo-controlled trial. Lancet 392(10163):2441–2451

van der Heijde D, Song IH, Pangan AL, Deodhar A, van den Bosch F, Maksymowych WP, Kim TH, Kishimoto M, Everding A, Sui Y, Wang X, Chu AD, Sieper J (2019) Efficacy and safety of upadacitinib in patients with active ankylosing spondylitis (SELECT-AXIS 1): a multicentre, randomised, double-blind, placebo-controlled, phase 2/3 trial. Lancet 394 (10214):2108–2117

Ward MM, Deodhar A, Akl EA et al (2016) American College of Rheumatology/Spondylitis Association of America/Spondyloarthritis Research and Treatment Network 2015 Recommendations for the Treatment of Ankylosing Spondylitis and Nonradiographic Axial Spondyloarthritis. Arthritis Rheumatol 68 (2):282–298

Ware JE Jr, Sherbourne CD (1992) The MOS 36-item short-form health survey (SF-36). I. Conceptual framework and item selection. Med Care 30(6):473–483

Yang X, Fan D, Xia Q, Wang M, Zhang X, Li X, Cai G, Wang L, Xin L, Xu S, Pan F (2016) The health-related quality of life of ankylosing spondylitis patients assessed by SF-36: a systematic review and meta-analysis. Qual Life Res 25(11):2711–2723

Zhu W, He X, Cheng K, Zhang L, Chen D, Wang X, Qiu G, Cao X, Weng X (2019) Ankylosing spondylitis: etiology, pathogenesis, and treatments. Bone Res 7(22)

Adv Exp Med Biol - Clinical and Experimental Biomedicine (2022) 13: 79–85
https://doi.org/10.1007/5584_2021_617

Published online: 10 March 2021

Changes of Motile Ciliary Phenotype in Patients with Primary Ciliopathies

Miroslava Brndiarova, Julia Kvassayova, Jarmila Vojtkova, Matus Igaz, Tomas Buday, and Jana Plevkova

Abstract

Primary ciliopathies are a group of disorders associated with abnormal formation and function of primary cilia. Many cilia-associated proteins found in primary cilia are also present in motile cilia. Such proteins are important for the ciliary base, such as the transition zone or basal bodies, and the intraflagellar transport. Their exact role in the respiratory motile cilia is unsettled. In this prospective clinical single-center study, we investigated the hypothesis that these proteins regulate the function of motile cilia. We addressed the issue by defining the motile cilia beat frequency in the respiratory tract of patients with primary ciliopathies accompanied by chronic kidney disease and comparing it in those without kidney involvement. Ciliary beat frequency in the nasal mucosa samples was evaluated by the ciliary analysis software LabVIEW. Both children and their parents with primary ciliopathies and kidney involvement had significantly lower median airway ciliary beat frequencies than those without kidney involvement who have normal ciliary motility. Further, the ciliary beat frequency is inversely associated with the serum creatinine level. These findings strongly suggest that kidney involvement in patients with primary ciliopathy may underlie the development of motile cilia dysfunction in the respiratory tract, potentially increasing respiratory morbidity.

Keywords

Cilia · Ciliary beat frequency · Ciliopathy · Kidney disease · Respiratory morbidity

1 Introduction

Cilia play a vital part in human physiology. They are divided into two main types. Motile cilia are found in the respiratory tract, ventricles of the central nervous system, and the middle ear. These cilia have a rhythmic beating motion and, for instance, in the respiratory tract, they are an important component of the airway defense by sweeping mucous out of the lungs (Kempeneers and Chilvers 2018). Primary cilia are nonmotile and typically appear on the apical surface of most eukaryotic cells as microtubule-based organelles covered with the plasma membrane. These cilia lack the two central microtubule singlets

M. Brndiarova (✉), J. Kvassayova, J. Vojtkova, and M. Igaz
Department of Pediatrics, Jessenius Faculty of Medicine and University Hospital, Comenius University in Bratislava, Martin, Slovakia
e-mail: brndiarova1@uniba.sk

T. Buday and J. Plevkova
Department of Pathophysiology, Jessenius Faculty of Medicine, Comenius University in Bratislava, Martin, Slovakia
e-mail: tomas.buday@uniba.sk; jana.plevkova@uniba.sk

characteristic of motile cilia. Primary cilia play an essential role for chemosensory (Bloodgood 2010), mechanosensory, for instance, detecting luminal flow in renal tubules, biliary ducts, and vessels (Nauli et al. 2003), and photosensory retinal functions (Senior et al. 1961). Primary ciliopathies are a group of disorders associated with abnormal formation and function of primary cilia. The clinical phenotypes of ciliopathy are diverse. A common feature of some primary ciliopathies is a variable extent of kidney damage or cyst formation (Braun and Hildebrandt 2017). Typical extra-renal manifestations include hepatic cysts and fibrosis (Schueler et al. 2015), retinal degeneration (Senior et al. 1961), skeletal deformities, dysmorphic facial features (Sensenbrenner et al. 1975), laterality defects, and congenital heart defects (Otto et al. 2003). Respiratory manifestations of primary ciliopathies like bronchiectasis, respiratory infection, or lung cysts are rare and their exact cause is unclear (Ibrahim and Rasoul 2015; Driscoll et al. 2008). Nonetheless, the respiratory tract is quite often affected by the disturbance of motile cilia manifest by impaired function of mucociliary clearance. The ciliary beating is coordinated in metachronal waves. It is a complex process that requires intertwined molecular interactions influenced by intracellular Ca^{2+} content and pH change, and protein kinase activation (Joskova et al. 2020; Marusiakova et al. 2020; Bayless et al. 2019; Duricek et al. 2019). Many cilia-associated proteins found in primary cilia are also present in motile cilia. Yet it is unclear to what extent proteins forming the ciliary basal body and the transition zone, and those engaged in the intraflagellar transport, could be concurrently affected in both types of cilia. Therefore, this study aims to evaluate the ciliary beat frequency (CBF) of the airway motile cilia in patients with a primary ciliopathy in an organ distal to the respiratory tract. We investigated the hypothesis that the airway CBF could be affected in primary ciliopathies involving kidneys, which would manifest in reduced airway mucus clearance. We addressed the issue by investigating the pediatric and adult (children's parents) patients with primary ciliopathies affecting kidneys.

2 Methods

2.1 Study Design and Population

This is a prospective clinical single-center study. We had four groups of patients: two each of children and adults with and without chronic kidney diseases, CKD(+) and CKD(−), respectively. Additionally, we had two groups of healthy age-matched children and adults with no kidney disease for the reference measurement of CBF. The group stratification with basic demographic data is shown in Table 1.

Inclusion criteria were the lack of acute respiratory infections in the preceding 4 weeks, no smoking, no allergy, and no use of antihistamines. The degree of chronic kidney disease (CKD) in adults was evaluated according to the National Kidney Foundation's CKD Epidemiology Collaboration (CKD-EPI) creatinine equation (Levey and Stevens 2010) and in children according to the bedside Schwartz equation (Schwartz and Work 2009). Basic demographic data, detailed respiratory history, laboratory indices data (plasma creatinine, urinalysis), abdominal ultrasonography, echocardiography, spirometry, and chest computer tomography were obtained from medical records. Exclusion criteria were adenoid hypertrophy, acute or chronic infections, and anatomical deformities identified during the ear-nose-throat examination.

Table 1 Stratification of study groups

	Primary ciliopathy—children		Primary ciliopathy—adults		Healthy children	Healthy adults
	CKD(+)	CKD(−)	CKD(+)	CKD(−)	CKD(−)	CKD(−)
n	3	16	3	5	43	21
Age (years)	14 (12–16)	9 (6–11)	54 (37–59)	37 (35–43)	10 (7–13)	42 (34–49)

Data are medians (IQR). *CDK(+)* chronic kidney disease, *CKD(−)* lack of chronic kidney disease, *n* number of subjects

Other exclusion criteria were gastroesophageal reflux disease, endocrine, metabolic, or oncological diseases.

2.2 Investigations

Samples of ciliated epithelium in nasal mucosa were obtained by a cytology brush (Cytobrush plus, Medscand Medical; CooperSurgical, Inc., Trumbull, CT) and suspended in the Roswell Park Memorial Institute (RPMI) 1640 medium. The temperature was maintained at 20 °C. Motile cilia were observed using a digital high-speed video camera (Basler A504kc; Basler AG; Ahrensburg, Germany) at a frame rate of 256–512 per sec. The camera was connected to an inverted phase-contrast microscope (Zeiss Axio Vert. A1; Carl Zeiss AG: Göttingen, Germany) and a computer. Specimens were examined using a 40× objective lens providing a magnification of 400×. Video analysis was performed using cilia analysis software (LabVIEW National Instruments Corp, Austin, TX) (Hargaš et al. 2011). Each preparation was evaluated for a maximum of 10 min, with 10 short video sequences recorded. The median and range of CBF were provided. Only undisrupted ciliated epithelia were analysed.

Genetic analysis was performed to confirm the presence of primary ciliopathy using the next-generation sequencing method using NextSeq System (Illumina Inc., San Diego, CA). The entire coding and splice-relevant regions of genes were evaluated.

2.3 Statistical Analysis

Data were expressed as medians and interquartile ranges (IQR). Differences were assessed using Student's *t*-test for unpaired samples. A *p*-value <0.05 defined statistically significant changes. The analysis was performed using a commercial SYSTAT v11.0 package (Systat Software Inc., San Jose, CA).

3 Results

3.1 Airway Ciliary Beat Frequency (CBF)—Motile Phenotype

The airway CBF in healthy children and their adult parents without primary ciliopathy and chronic kidney diseases was, on average, between 6 and 8 Hz and was alike in both groups as detailed in Table 2. This value of CBF was taken as a reference level for comparison to that in patients with primary ciliopathies and chronic kidney involvement. Children and their parents with CKD had the median airway CBF, on average, between 4 and 5 Hz, which was a highly significant decline compared to the patients without CKD ($p < 0.001$). There were no appreciable differences in CBF between the two age groups of patients in the presence or absence of CKD (Table 3). The CBF in patients without CKD was at the level of that present in the control healthy subjects.

Table 2 Airway ciliary beat frequency in healthy control subjects without primary ciliopathy and chronic kidney diseases (CKD−)

	CKD(−)
Ciliary beat frequency (Hz)	
Children	6.7 (6.0–7.7)
Adults	6.2 (5.3–7.3)
p (children/adult)	> 0.05
Creatinine (μmol/l)	
Children	55 (47–66)
Adults	73 (67–79)
p (children/adult)	0.03

Data are medians (IQR)

Table 3 Airway ciliary beat frequency and serum creatinine level in patients with and without chronic kidney diseases, CKD(+) and CKD(−), respectively

	CKD (+)	CKD (−)	*p*
Ciliary beat frequency (Hz)			
Children	4.0 (3.9–4.8)	6.8 (6.5–7.1)	< 0.0001
Adults	4.9 (4.3–5.0)	6.9 (6.7–7.1)	< 0.001
p (children/adult)	0.45	0.39	
Creatinine (μmol/l)			
Children	296 (225–299)	57 (47–78)	0.00003
Adults	216 (186–315)	62 (47–81)	0.003
p (children/adult)	0.43	0.39	

Data are medians (IQR)

3.2 Respiratory Manifestations

Respiratory manifestations were seen in 100% of children with CKD(+) and 6.3% of children with CKD(−). Concerning the adult patients, respiratory manifestations were seen in 33.3% with CKD(+) and in none with CKD(−). Patients with nephronophthisis type I (NPHP type 1) did not suffer from respiratory infections but had a restrictive lung disorder and nonspecific nodules up to 5 mm in diameter in the upper lobes of lung parenchyma (segments: S10 bilateral and S6 in the right lung). Overall, a restrictive lung disorder was seen in 50% of patients with CKD. A 10-year-old boy with Sensenbrenner syndrome (SBS) and low CBF had mild recurrent rhinosinusitis. Two patients with autosomal recessive polycystic kidney disease (ARPKD) had recurrent rhinitis. One of them belonged to the CKD(+) group and had a strongly decreased lower CBF of 3.8 (3.2–6.0) Hz. Another CKD(+) patient with the autosomal dominant polycystic kidney disease (ADPKD) and a restrictive lung disorder also had a low CBF of 3.8 (3.2–5.9) Hz. Computer tomography of the lungs did not detect bronchiectasis in the patients.

3.3 Genetic Analysis

The presence of primary kidney ciliopathy was confirmed in the genetic analysis. We found that patients with ADPKD commonly had a mutation in the *PKD1* gene (88.0%). We identified 6 new pathogenic variants of this gene found in 11 patients (Table 4).

4 Discussion

This study demonstrates that patients with primary ciliopathies with developed CKD had reduced ciliary beating frequency in the airway mucosal cells. The most likely underlying reason could be an impaired ciliary structure caused by mutations of the genes encoding ciliary proteins that are identical for both primary and motile cilia. Several hypotheses of the origin of respiratory manifestations in patients with primary kidney ciliopathies are presented in the literature. One of them is a disorder of calcium homeostasis leading to reduced cellular calcium signaling in patients with polycystic kidney diseases. Calcium plays a critical role in regulating CBF (Mangolini et al. 2016; Nauli et al. 2003; Braiman and Priel 2001). Wu et al. (2009) have suggested that damage to primary cilia in airway smooth muscle cells could underlie motile cilia dysfunction. Bronchiectases are frequently associated with irregular bronchial wall thickness. Primary cilia of airway smooth muscle cells may be mechanical pressure sensors and play a role in cell migration, injury repair, and possibly in ciliogenesis. Motile ciliated cells originate from primary ciliated cells. When ciliogenesis is impaired, cilia exhibit slow and dyskinetic motion (Jain et al. 2010). An unresolved question is whether the sensory function of primary cilia is also present in motile cilia (Jain et al. 2012).

The present findings are comparable to those of Shoemark et al. (2015) who have found that patients with Bardet-Biedl syndrome have normal CBF. Likewise, Fliegauf et al. (2006) have found that in the absence of nephrocystin, a molecular

Table 4 Pathogenic mutations in the *PKD1* gene that encodes the protein polycystin-1 active in kidney primary cilia. Individual subjects, renal and extrarenal manifestations, as well as the patients' airway ciliary beat frequency (CBF) are shown. New pathogenic mutations unraveled are bold out

Sex	Mutation/gene	CBF (Hz)	Renal manifestations	Extrarenal manifestations
F	*PKHD1*	3.8	CKD G4, HT, P	Hepatic cysts and fibrosis, respiratory infections
M	*PKHD1*	6.5	HT	Hepatic cysts, respiratory infections
F	*PKHD1*	7.1		
F	*PKHD1*	6.0	HT	Hepatic fibrosis
F	***PKD1* c.2528C > G, p.(Ser843*) exon 11**	9.0		
M	***PKD1* c.7525_7539dup, p. (Val2509_Leu2513dup)**	8.3		
M	***PKD1* c.11425G > C, p. (Gly3809_Arg)**	8.7		
F	*PKD1*	7.0		
M	***PKD1* c.3114delA, p.(Leu1039*)**	7.0		
M	***PKD1* c.3400_3401delArg(p. Ser1134)**	6.4		
M	***PKD1* c.3400_3401delArg(p. Ser1134)**	6.9		
F	***PKD1* c9683dupG, p. (Leu3229Profs*24) exon 28**	6.7		
F	*PKD2*	6.6		
F	*PKD2*	7.2		
F	*PKD1*	3.0	CKD G4, HT, P	Hepatic cysts, restrictive lung disorder
F	*PKD1*	4.9	CKD G3b, HT, P	Hepatic cysts
M	*PKD1*	5.0	CKD, G3a, HT	
M	***PKD1* c.3400_3401delAG(p. Ser1134)**	6.7	HT	
M	*PKD1*	7.1		
F	*PKD2*	6.2	HT, P	Hepatic cysts
F	*PKD1*	6.9		
M	***PKD1* c.3114delA, p.(Leu1039*)**	7.9		
F	*NPHP1 (homozygote)*	4.0	CKD G5, P, HT, Tx	LVNC, nonspecific lung nodules, restrictive lung disorder
M	***WDR35* c.1922 T > G, p.(Leu641*), c.2522A > Tp.(Asp841Val)**	5.6	CKD G3b, HT, P	Foramen ovale, hypospadias, Cranioectodermal dysplasia, respiratory infections
M	***WDR35* c.1922 T > G, p.(Leu641*), c.2522A > Tp.(Asp841Val)**	6.5		Cranioectodermal dysplasia
M	*BBS9*	6.7		Syndactyly, Hirschsprung disease, hypogonadism
F	OFD type I	6.5		Syndactyly, brachydactyly

CKD chronic kidney disease, *Arg* arginine, *Asp* aspartate, *BBS* Bardet-Biedl syndrome, *Gly* glycine, *HT* hypertension, *Leu* leucine, *LVNC* left ventricular non-compaction cardiomyopathy, *OFD type I* orofaciodigital syndrome, *P* proteinuria, *Ser* serine, *Tx* kidney transplantation, *Val* valine

component of primary cilia, the structure of motile cilia remains unaltered, and the CBF is normal. The beating pattern may be slightly irregular, but the irregularity is not as severe as in primary ciliary dyskinesia. Therefore, the presumption that proteins that regulate ciliary motion would be damaged in patients with primary ciliopathies is hardly tenable.

Ciliopathies are a heterogeneous group of disorders. Phenotypic features are variable even in patients with the same mutations. Walczak-Sztulpa et al. (2017) have reported the intrafamilial variability in patients with Sensenbrenner syndrome with heterozygous variants in the *WDR35* gene. We observed two female siblings with ciliopathies having different phenotypic features (these two patients were not included in the present study group; unpublished observation). One girl had polycystic kidney disease. Her renal function was normal and the CBF remained in the normal range of 7.2 (6.5–8.4) Hz. The other girl had the CBF significantly reduced down to the level of 1.1 (0–2) Hz characteristic of primary ciliary dyskinesia. This girl had a normal renal function and no cystic kidney formations but suffered from recurrent respiratory infections. The plausibility is that the siblings had different clinical manifestations of the same cilia-elated disorder. However, the varied expression of relevant genes or genetic mutations ("genetic load") that can modulate clinical manifestation cannot be excluded (Arts and Knoers 2013; Bredrup et al. 2011).

It is generally known that patients with CKD are more likely to experience respiratory manifestations (Pierson 2006). A cross-sectional study of Kucur et al. (2016) who used saccharin tests suggests that chronic kidney failure is a risk for respiratory mucociliary dysfunction. According to that study, nasal mucociliary clearance time is significantly greater in patients with CKD than in healthy control individuals. No studies have yet directly evaluated the respiratory CBF in patients with kidney failure. There are several potential mechanisms of damage to respiratory cilia in this condition like free oxygen radicals or uremic toxins, endothelial dysfunction and vasoconstriction with reduced blood flow, decreased periciliary fluid flow, or increased mucus viscosity with electrolyte imbalance (Uluyol et al. 2016). The design of the present study did not make it possible to distinguish the exact molecular mechanism of respiratory cilia dysfunction. Yet we believe we have shown that motile cilia in the airways of patients with CKD are defunct as expressed by significantly reduced CBF. Further, we submit that genetic factors and disturbed body homeostasis in CKD may impair mucociliary transport function in the airways of patients with primary ciliopathies.

Conflicts of Interest The authors declare no conflicts of interest in relation to this study.

Ethical Approval All procedures performed in studies involving human participants were in accord with the ethical standards of the institutional and/or national research committee and with the 1964 Helsinki declaration and its later amendments or comparable ethical standards.

Informed Consent Informed consent was obtained from all individual participants included in the study.

References

Arts HH, Knoers NV (2013) Current insights into renal ciliopathies: what can genetics teach us? Pediatr Nephrol 28(6):863–874

Bayless BA, Navarro FM, Winey M (2019) Motile cilia: innovation and insight from ciliate model organisms. Front Cell Dev Biol 7:265

Bloodgood RA (2010) Sensory reception is an attribute of both primary cilia and motile cilia. J Cell Sci 123 (pt 4):505–509

Braiman A, Priel Z (2001) Intracellular stores maintain stable cytosolic Ca^{2+} gradients in epithelial cells by active Ca^{2+} redistribution. Cell Calcium 30 (6):361–371

Braun DA, Hildebrandt F (2017) Ciliopathies. Cold Spring Harb Perspect Biol 9(3):a028191

Bredrup C, Saunier S, Oud MM et al (2011) Ciliopathies with skeletal anomalies and renal insufficiency due to mutations in the IFT-A gene WDR19. Am J Hum Genet 89(5):634–643

Driscoll JA, Bhalla S, Liapis H, Ibricevic A, Brody SL (2008) Autosomal dominant polycystic kidney disease is associated with an increased prevalence of radiographic bronchiectasis. Chest 133(5):1181–1188

Duricek M, Banovcin P, Halickova T, Hyrdel R, Kollarik M (2019) Acidic pharyngeal reflux does not correlate with symptoms and laryngeal injury attributed to laryngopharyngeal reflux. Dig Dis Sci 64 (5):1270–1280

Fliegauf M, Horvath J, von Schnakenburg C, Olbrich H, Müller D, Thumfart J, Schermer B, Pazour GJ, Neumann HP, Zentgraf H, Benzing T, Omran H (2006) Nephrocystin specifically localizes to the transition zone of renal and respiratory cilia and photoreceptor connecting cilia. J Am Soc Nephrol 17(9):2424–2433

Hargaš L, Koniar D, Štofan S (2011) Sophisticated biomedical tissue measurement using image analysis and virtual instrumentation. In: Folea S (ed) Practical applications and solutions using LabVIEW™ Software. InTech, Rijeka, pp 155–180

Ibrahim WH, Rasoul FA (2015) Pulmonary manifestations of adult polycystic kidney disease: case report and literature review. Ibnosina J Med Biomed Sci 7 (5):169–172

Jain R, Pan J, Driscoll JA, Wisner JW, Huang T, Gunsten SP, You Y, Brody SL (2010) Temporal relationship between primary and motile ciliogenesis in airway epithelial cells. Am J Respir Cell Mol Biol 43(6):731–739

Jain R, Javidan-Nejad C, Alexander-Brett J, Horani A, Cabellon MC, Walter MJ, Brody SL (2012) Sensory functions of motile cilia and implication for bronchiectasis. Front Biosci (Schol Ed) 4:1088–1099

Joskova M, Durdik P, Sutovska M, Grendar M, Koniar D, Hargas L, Banovcin P, Franova S (2020) Negative impact of anesthesia with midazolam, sufentanil, and propofol used in pediatric flexible bronchoscopy on the tracheal ciliary beat frequency in guinea pigs. J Pharmacol Sci 142(4):165–171

Kempeneers C, Chilvers MA (2018) To beat, or not to beat, that is question! The spectrum of ciliopathies. Pediatr Pulmonol 53(8):1122–1129

Kucur C, Ozbay I, Gulcan E, Kulekci S, Aksoy S, Oghan F (2016) Evaluation of nasal mucociliary activity in patients with chronic renal failure. Eur Arch Otorhinolaryngol 273(5):1167–1171

Levey AS, Stevens LA (2010) Estimating GFR using the CKD epidemiology collaboration (CKD-EPI) creatinine equation: more accurate GFR estimates, lower CKD prevalence estimates, and better risk predictions. Am J Kidney Dis 55(4):622–627

Mangolini A, de Stephanis L, Aguiari G (2016) Role of calcium in polycystic kidney disease: from signaling to pathology. World J Nephrol 5(1):76–83

Marusiakova L, Durdik P, Jesenak M, Bugova G, Kvassayova J, Oppova D, Banovcin P (2020) Ciliary beat frequency in children with adenoid hypertrophy. Pediatr Pulmonol 55(3):666–673

Nauli SM, Alenghat FJ, Luo Y, Williams E, Vassilev P, Li X, Elia AE, Lu W, Brown EM, Quinn SJ, Ingber DE, Zhou J (2003) Polycystins 1 and 2 mediate mechanosensation in the primary cilium of kidney cells. Nat Genet 33(2):129–137

Otto EA, Schermer B, Obara T et al (2003) Mutations in INVS encoding inversion cause nephronophthisis type 2, linking renal cystic disease to the function of primary cilia and left-right axis determination. Nat Genet 34(4):413–420

Pierson JD (2006) Respiratory considerations in the patient with renal failure. Respir Care 51(4):413–422

Schueler M, Braun DA, Chandrasekar G et al (2015) DCDC2 mutations cause a renal-hepatic ciliopathy by disrupting Wnt signaling. Am J Hum Genet 96 (1):81–92

Schwartz GJ, Work DF (2009) Measurement and estimation of GFR in children and adolescents. J Am Soc Nephrol 4(11):1832–1643

Senior B, Friedmann AI, Braudo JL (1961) Juvenile familial nephropathy with tapetoretinal degeneration: a new oculorenal dystrophy. Am J Ophthalmol 52:625–633

Sensenbrenner JA, Dorst JP, Owens RP (1975) New syndrome of skeletal, dental and hair anomalies. Birth Defects Orig Artic Ser 11(2):372–379

Shoemark A, Dixon M, Beales PL, Hogg CL (2015) Bardet Biedl syndrome: motile ciliary phenotype. Chest 147(3):764–770

Uluyol S, ALP A, Kilicaslan S, Gur MH (2016) Nasal mucociliary clearance in chronic renal failure: comparison of pre-dialysis and dialysis stages. Tepecik Eğit Hast Derg 26:197–200

Walczak-Sztulpa J, Wawrocka A, Sobierajewicz A, Kuszel L, Zawadzki J, Grenda R, Swiader-Lesniak A, Kocyla-Karczmarewicz B, Wnuk A, Latos-Bielenska-A, Chrzanowska KH (2017) Intrafamilial phenotypic variability in a Polish family with Sensenbrenner syndrome and biallelic WDR35 mutations. Am J Med Genet A 173(5):1364–1368

Wu J, Du H, Wang X, Mei CH, Sieck GC, Qian Q (2009) Characterization of primary cilia in human airway smooth muscle cells. Chest 136(2):561–570

Adv Exp Med Biol - Clinical and Experimental Biomedicine (2022) 13: 87–101
https://doi.org/10.1007/5584_2021_633

Published online: 20 March 2021

Effects of Inhalation of STIM-Orai Antagonist SKF 96365 on Ovalbumin-Induced Airway Remodeling in Guinea Pigs

Martina Šutovská, Michaela Kocmálová, Ivana Kazimierová, Christina Imnoy Nøss Forsberg, Marta Jošková, Marian Adamkov, and Soňa Fraňová

Abstract

Airway remodeling (AR) consists of wall thickening and hyperreactivity. STIM (stromal interaction molecule) and Orai protein pathways mediate extracellular Ca^{2+} signals involved in AR. This study aims to define the effects on AR of the STIM-Orai antagonist SKF 96365 given by inhalation in three increasing doses in ovalbumin-induced AR. In the control group, the antiasthmatic budesonide and salbutamol were given in the same model. The airway structure was evaluated by histological and immunohistochemistry and reactivity by specific airway resistance, contraction strength of isolated airway smooth muscles, and mucociliary clearance expressed by ciliary beating frequency. The immuno-biochemical markers of chronic inflammation were evaluated by BioPlex and ELISA assays. The AR was mediated by inflammatory cytokines and growth factors. The findings show significant anti-remodeling effects of SKF 96365, which were associated with a decrease in airway hyperreactivity. The anti-remodeling effect of SKF 96365 was mediated via the suppression of IL-4, IL-5, and IL-13 synthesis, and IL-12–INF-γ–TGF-β pathway. The budesonide-related AR suppression had to do with a decrease in proinflammatory cytokines and an increase in the anti-inflammatory IL-10, with negligible influence on growth factors synthesis and mucous glands activity.

Keywords

Airway hyperactivity · Airway remodeling · Biomarkers · Cytokines · Inflammation · SKF 96365 · STIM-Orai pathway

M. Šutovská, C. I. N. Forsberg, M. Jošková, and S. Fraňová
Department of Pharmacology, Jessenius Faculty of Medicine, Comenius University, Mala Hora, Martin, Slovakia
e-mail: martina.sutovska@uniba.sk; forsberg1@uniba.sk; marta.joskova@uniba.sk; sona.franova@uniba.sk

M. Kocmálová (✉) and I. Kazimierová
Department of Pharmacology, Jessenius Faculty of Medicine, Comenius University, Mala Hora, Martin, Slovakia

Martin's Biomedical Center (BioMed), Jessenius Faculty of Medicine, Comenius University, Martin, Slovakia
e-mail: michaela.kocmalova@uniba.sk; kocmalova@jfmed.uniba.sk; ivana.kazimierova@gmail.com

M. Adamkov
Institute of Histology and Embryology Jessenius Faculty of Medicine Comenius University, Martin, Slovakia
e-mail: adamkov@uniba.sk

1 Introduction

Airway remodeling (AR) refers to structural changes resulting from repeated injury and repair processes. The AR in asthma consists of epithelial alterations and metaplasia, increased deposition of extracellular matrix components under the bronchial subepithelial basement membrane (Boulet 2018), airway smooth muscle (ASM) hypertrophy and hyperplasia (Munakata 2006), gland enlargement, and neovascularization (Bergeron et al. 2010). Immunologic and molecular mechanisms that drive the progression of asthma to AR are still incompletely understood. Studies of allergen-induced AR in transgenic mice suggest roles for cytokines, chemokines, and growth factors, such as transforming growth factor-beta (TGF-β), vascular endothelial growth factor (VEGF), Th_2 cytokines—interleukin-5 (IL-5), IL-9, and IL-13, and epithelial-derived nuclear factor kappa B (NF-κB)-regulated chemokines (Doherty and Broide 2007). The release of TGF-β by injured epithelium results in the synthesis of extracellular matrix proteins by fibroblasts and myofibroblasts (Hostettler et al. 2008) and secretion of cytokines, chemokines, and growth factors by modulating autocrine proliferative responses of ASM, all of which driving the AR (Spinelli et al. 2012; Shore 2002). Some other cytokines affecting airway inflammation or structural cells such as tumor necrosis factor-alpha (TNF-α), IL-4, fibroblast growth factor (FGF), or epidermal growth factor (EGF) also have this potential (Busse et al. 2005; Kuperman et al. 2005).

Growth factors acting via tyrosine kinase receptors, inflammatory mediators, like histamine, acting via G protein-coupled receptors, and cytokines acting via cell surface glycoprotein receptors increase the cytoplasmic content of calcium ions (Ca^{2+}). A rise in Ca^{2+}, besides contraction and proliferation of ASM, mediates mucus production, ciliary beat frequency, or cytokine/chemokine synthesis in structural and inflammatory cells. A major conduit for Ca^{2+} influx in non-excitable cells is through plasma membrane store-operated channels (SOC) (Samanta and Parekh 2016) following the emptying of Ca^{2+} stores in the endoplasmic reticulum. In immune cells, calcium release-activated channels (CRAC), containing stromal interaction molecule (STIM) and Orai proteins in the endoplasmic reticulum, activate de novo synthesis and secretion of pro-inflammatory leukotrienes and increase expressions of c-Fos, nuclear factor of activated T-cells (NFAT), and various cytokines which orchestrate the subsequent inflammatory responses (Sutovska et al. 2016; Hogan et al. 2010; Vig et al. 2008). SOC-mediated Ca^{2+} entry also is involved in TGF-β-facilitated ASM cell proliferation (Gao et al. 2013) and IL-13/TNF-α induced airway hyperresponsiveness (Spinelli and Trebak 2016; Jia et al. 2013). The ASM remodeling in asthma is associated with changes in the expression of ion channels and pumps (Mahn et al. 2010; Perez-Zoghbi et al. 2009). The ASM cells from asthmatic mice display an increased expression of STIM-Orai proteins (Spinelli et al. 2012).

Targeting CRAC channels seems a promising approach to managing chronic airway diseases. The combined modulation of airway epithelial, ASM, and inflammatory cell activities by CRAC channel inhibitors could effectively dampen airway hyperreactivity, inflammatory, and remodeling components. We investigated this hypothesis in the present study in an experimental model of ovalbumin-induced airway remodeling in the guinea pig.

2 Methods

2.1 Animals

A total of 70 adult guinea pigs, strain TRIK, weighing 150–300 g were used in the study. The animals were obtained from the Department of Experimental Pharmacology of the Slovak Academy of Sciences, in Dobra Voda, Slovakia, and underwent at least one-week adaptation period in the animal house, having commercial chow and water ad libitum. Additionally, they were adapted to the laboratory environment for several days before experiments, with the ambient temperature of 21–24 °C and relative humidity of 55 ± 10%. There were 7 randomly selected groups consisting of 10 animals each. The airway inflammation was induced in six groups, with the remaining group serving as a healthy ovalbumin-negative (OVA-) control. All the remaining animals were sensitized by repetitive administration of the OVA allergen for 28 days. From the 14th day of sensitization on, the treatment by salmeterol, budesonide, and SKF 96365 (1-[2-(4-Methoxyphenyl)-2-[3-(4-methoxyphenyl) propoxy]ethyl-1*H*-imidazole hydrochloride) was started in five experimental groups. The sixth group, OVA28, was exposed only to isotonic saline (5 min inhalations) and served as a sensitized negative control group. SKF 96365 groups were exposed for 5 min to different doses/concentrations of the compound by the inhalation route: SKF2.5 – 2.5 μM, SKF5.0 – 5.0 μM, and SKF10 – 10 μM. The tested SKF 96365 compound and two control drugs, salmeterol (SAL – 0.17 mM, 5 min inhalation) and budesonide (BUD – 1 mM, 5 min inhalation), were applied once daily for 14 days. The influence of SKF 96365 on airway defense mechanisms was evaluated in all three concentration groups receiving it. The immunohistochemistry was performed on specimens taken from the group of animals treated with the highest SKF 96365 concentration of 10 μM having the most pronounced effects.

2.2 Reagents

Chicken ovalbumin, histamine, salmeterol, and budesonide were purchased from Sigma-Aldrich (Bratislava, Slovakia), SKF 96365 from Tocris Bioscience (Bristol, Great Britain), aluminum hydroxide and Tween 80 from Centralchem (Bratislava, Slovakia), methacholine and saline (sodium chloride solution) from ApliChem (Darmstadt, Germany), RPMI 1640 medium from Gibco/Thermo Fisher Scientific (Waltham, MA).

SKF 96365 and salmeterol were dissolved in water for injection, budesonide in 1% Tween 80, and all other chemicals in saline. Solutions of all compounds were aerosolized by a PARI jet nebulizer (output 5 L/s, particles mass median diameter 1.2 μm; Paul Ritzau, Pari-Werk GmbH, Starnberg, Germany) and delivered to the head-out plethysmograph composed of separate nasal and body chambers (HSE type 855; Hugo Sachs Electronic, March, Germany) where the animals were placed. The experimental procedures were accomplished 24 h after the last drug application.

2.3 Ovalbumin Sensitization and Challenge Protocol

For the 28-day long sensitization, OVA adsorbed on aluminum hydroxide in saline, 5 mg OVA, and 100 mg $Al(OH)_3$ was administered parenterally as follows: Day 1 intraperitoneally and subcutaneously, Day 4 intraperitoneally, and Day 12 subcutaneously. Afterward, it was nebulized and the mist was introduced into the head chamber of a plethysmograph at Days 9, 15, 18, 20, 24, and 27. The OVA(−) group of animals (healthy negative control) was challenged for 28 days with isotonic saline only.

2.4 Morphology and Immunohistochemistry

Airway Reactivity In Vivo Specific airway resistance (sRaw) was used to evaluate the airway reactivity in vivo, mostly expressing the contractility of ASM cells. Conscious guinea pigs were individually placed in the head-out body plethysmograph. sRaw was calculated according to Pennock et al.'s (1979) method based on the airflow difference between the two chambers of the body plethysmograph. Changes in sRaw were recorded for 1 min after 30-s long histamine (10^{-5} M) and methacholine (10^{-5} M) inhalation. There was a 1 min interval between inhalations of bronchoconstrictor, with fresh air blowing into the head chamber.

Ciliary Beat Frequency (CBF) In Vitro A specimen of the ciliated epithelium was brush-taken from the trachea for an in vitro investigation. The temperature of the nutritive RPMI 1640 medium for cilia was maintained at 37–38 °C using a PeCon Temp Controller 2000–2 (PeCon GmbH; Erbach, Germany). Specimens were put onto glass slides and evaluated under an inverted phase-contrast microscope (Zeiss Axio Vert. A1; Carl Zeiss AG; Jena, Germany). Impaired ciliated cells were discarded. Sequential 10-s video files were recorded at 1 min intervals for 15 min at a frame rate from 256 to 512 frames/s using a digital high-speed video camera (Basler A504kc; Basler AG; Ahrensburg, Germany). The CBF was evaluated using Ciliary Analysis software (LabVIEW™) to generate a ciliary region of interest (ROI) (Hargas et al. 2011).

Histological and Immunohistochemical (IHC) Analysis Histomorphological and IHC staining was performed on formalin-fixed paraffin-embedded tissue samples collected from guinea pigs' left lungs, serially cut at 4 μm thickness. Gömöri's staining was used for reticulin fibers, anti-alpha smooth muscle actin (SMA), and anti-mucin 5 AC (MUC5AC) antibodies (Abcam; Cambridge, UK) for immunohistochemistry. To achieve a better adherence of tissue sections for immunoreactions, we used silanized slides (DAKO; Glostrup, Denmark), which were baked for 2 h in an oven at 59 °C. Immunohistochemical staining was performed by the autostainer BenchMark ULTRA (Roche; Rotkreuz, Switzerland) with mouse monoclonal antibodies MUC5AC (MRQ 19 clone, the incubation time of 16 min) and SMA (1A4 clone, the incubation time of 28 min) using Kit ultraView DAB (Ventana Medical Systems Inc.; Munich, Germany). All sections were counterstained with hematoxylin (DAKO, Glostrup, Denmark). For negative controls, the primary antibody was omitted. Slides were viewed under the Olympus BX41 microscope (Olympus; Tokyo, Japan). The image capture and the measurement of the thickness of bronchi walls (μm) in 10–15 similar size random bronchi in each section were performed using Quick Photo Micro software v2.2 (Olympus, Tokyo, Japan). The degree of MUC5AC positivity was semi-quantitatively determined by two independent observers under a dual-head microscope and grading system as previously described (Sutovska et al. 2015). Each specimen processed was evaluated as negative (degree 0 and 1) or positive (degree 2 and 3).

2.5 Biochemistry

Cytokines Animals were killed by transversal interruption of the cervical spinal cord and respiratory tract organs were removed. Bronchoalveolar lavage (BALF) was obtained by application of 10 mL/kg of 0.9% saline at 37 °C BBC Breaking News @BBCBreaking· Mar 4 Prince Philip has had "successful procedure" for pre-existing heart condition and will stay in hospital for number of days, Buckingham Palace says into a ligated left lung. The supernatant was acquired by centrifugation at 1500 rpm for 2 min. The Bio-Plex® 200 System and Bio-Plex Pro™ Human Cytokine Th1/Th2 Assay (Bio-Rad, Hercules, CA) were used to assess the content of cytokines and chemokines involved with the allergic inflammation of airways, such as IL-4, IL-5, IL-10, IL-12, IL-13, TNF-α, granulocyte-macrophage colony-stimulating factor (GM-CSF), and interferon-gamma (INF-γ). The assay is based on the sandwich ELISA design using magnetic beads. The measured analyte is bound between the capture and detection antibodies. The capture antibody-coupled beads were first incubated with antigen standards, samples, or controls, followed by the incubation with biotinylated detection antibodies and the reporter streptavidin-phycoerythrin (S-P) conjugate. Then, the beads were passed through the Bio-Plex 200 suspension array reader, equipped with two lasers of 532 nm and 635 nm excitations to measure the fluorescence of beads and bound S-P. A high-speed digital processor managed the data output, and the Bio-Plex Manager™ v6.0 software presented the concentration results in pg/mL.

Enzyme-Linked Immunosorbent Assay (ELISA) and Specific Reagents Supernatants from BALF and lung tissue homogenates were used for the quantification of growth factors. Lung tissue homogenates were prepared by sonication with a power output of 700 W (Stuart homogenizer in

SHM/STAND; Ecomed, Bratislava, Slovakia) in 1 mL of lysis solution (Tissue Extraction Reagent I Invitrogen™, ThermoFisher Scientific, Waltham, MA) containing a protease inhibitor cocktail (Sigma Aldrich Chemicals, St. Louis, MO). Samples were centrifuged at 10,000 rpm for 5 min at 4 °C (MICRO 220R Centrifuge, Hettich GmbH, Tuttlingen, Germany). BALF and homogenate supernatants were collected into sterile tubes and frozen at −80 °C for further analysis.

The level of TGF-β was determined in the supernatant from lung homogenates using an ELISA kit for transforming growth factor beta-1 (USCN Life Science Inc., Houston, TX) and EGF in the BALF supernatant using a kit for guinea pig total epidermal growth factor (MyBioSource, San Diego, CA) according to the manufacturer's instructions. The absorbance was measured spectrophotometrically at a wavelength of 450 nm and output data were assessed by SkanIt Software for Varioskan® Flash v2.4.5 (ThermoFisher Scientific, Waltham, MA). The detection levels were 5.7 pg /mL for TGF-β and 0.1 ng/mL for EGF.

2.6 Statistical Elaboration

Data on cytokines, growth factors, and sRaw were expressed as means ±SE. Data on the thickness of the SMA/collagen III layer were expressed as medians of representative 12–15 bronchial walls assessed in each guinea pig. CBFs were expressed as a median value (Hz) for each ROI, followed by the calculation of the arithmetic mean in each microscopic preparation. Student's *t*-test or one-way ANOVA with *post-hoc* Bonferroni test was selected as appropriate to test for statistically significant intergroup differences. Fisher's exact test was selected to evaluate the findings in the immunohistochemical analysis of MUC5AC. A p-value <0.05 defined significant differences. The analysis was performed using a commercial statistical package of GraphPad Prism software v6.01 (San Diego, CA).

3 Results

3.1 Effects of SKF 96365 on Airway Defense Mechanisms

Specific Airway Resistance (sRaw) Consistent with the histomorphological part of the study that clearly showed an increase in the ASM mass in the OVA28 group, there were significant differences in the basal, histamine-induced, and methacholine-induced sRaw when compared to OVA(−) group (Fig. 1). In vivo contractility of airways, whether in basal conditions or induced by either bronchoconstrictor, was significantly reduced in all experimental, with SKF 96365, and positive control, with salmeterol, groups of guinea pigs. SKF 96365 is a nonspecific SOC inhibitor causing effective and relatively selective CRAC channel inhibition when it is used in a concentration from 2 μM (Singh et al. 2010) to 12 μM (Spinelli and Trebak 2016; Chung et al. 1994), and salmeterol is a well-known classic asthma reliever. The CRAC channel blocker showed a dose-dependent suppression of mediator-induced airway hyperreactivity. Further, 14-day-long daily inhalation of 10 μM SKF 96365 exceeded the impact of the long-acting β-agonist salmeterol.

Ciliary Beating Frequency (CBF) We assessed the CBF as a key determinant of inflammation-induced AR in the ovalbumin-sensitized animals and the influence of CRAC channel inhibition on mucociliary clearance. The AR was associated with a negligible decrease in CBF. However, long-term treatment by SKF 96365 in the lowest tested concentration of 2.5 μM significantly inhibited the motion of cilia, as opposed to the control drugs budesonide and salmeterol or SKF 96365 in higher doses, all of which did not further suppress the CBF (Fig. 2).

Morphological Features of Airways Immunohistology was used to evaluate lung tissue specimens for the inflammation-induced structural changes in the ovalbumin-sensitized animals and the subsequent effects of long-term treatment

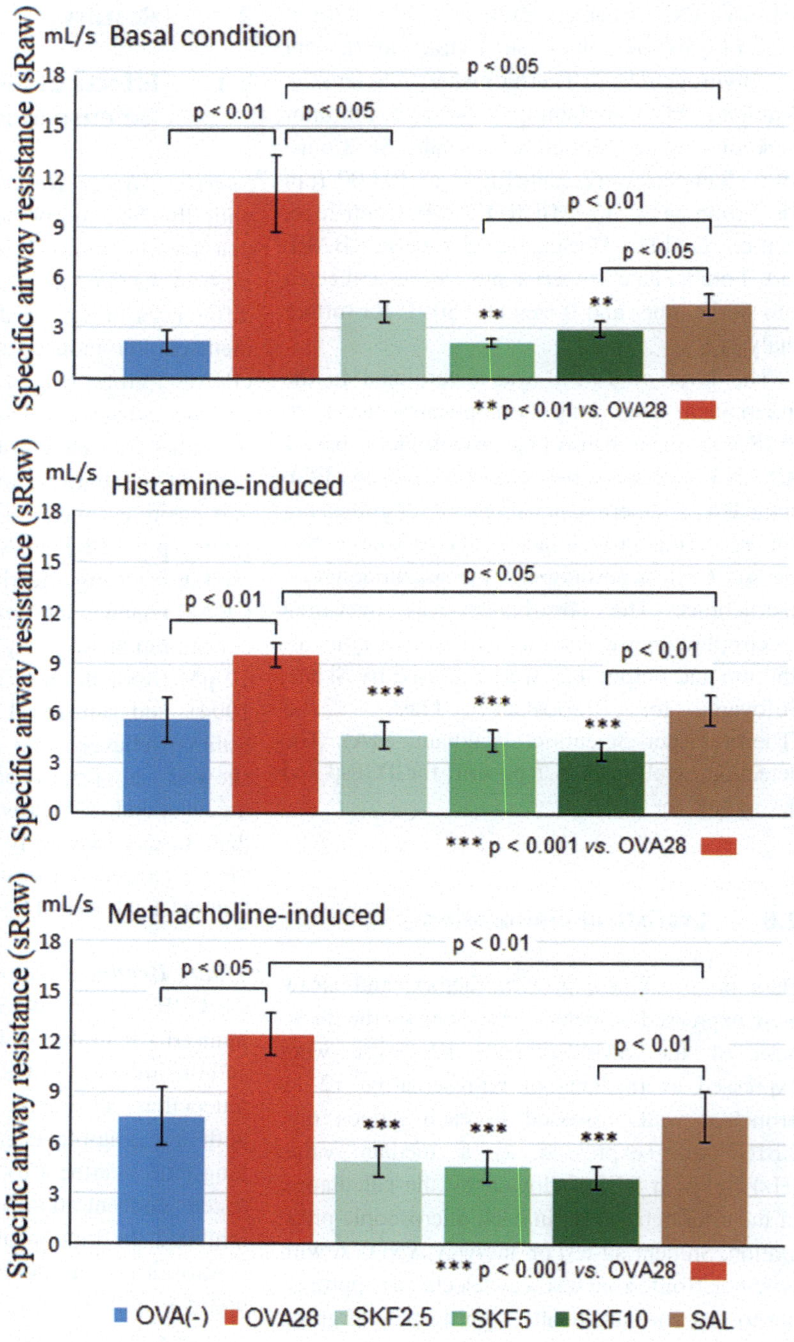

Fig. 1 Effects of inhalation of SKF 96365 in increasing concentrations on airway hyperreactivity assessed from the contractile response on the background of the ovalbumin (OVA)-sensitized guinea pigs. Top panel—basal condition—OVA sensitization and inhalations of isotonic saline only; middle panel—histamine inhalation in OVA-sensitized animals; bottom panel—methacholine inhalation in OVA-sensitized animals. The contractile response was expressed as the specific airway resistance (sRaw). OVA(−), unsensitized control; OVA28, sensitized negative control group; SKF2.5, 5, and 10 sensitized and treated with inhalation of SKF 96365 in the successively doubled concentrations of 2.5, 5, and 10 μM; and SAL, sensitized positive control group treated with inhalation of beta-2 agonist salmeterol (one-way ANOVA and post hoc Bonferroni test)

by the highest concentration of SKF 96365 as well as the classical corticosteroid anti-asthmatic budesonide. For comparison, specimens from saline-exposed animals were used (OVA-). Specimens from the sensitized negative controls (OVA28) showed the remodeling features such as subepithelial fibrosis, goblet cell hyperplasia, and increased ASM mass (Fig. 3). These changes were partially reverted in specimens from both SKF 96365 and budesonide-treated animals.

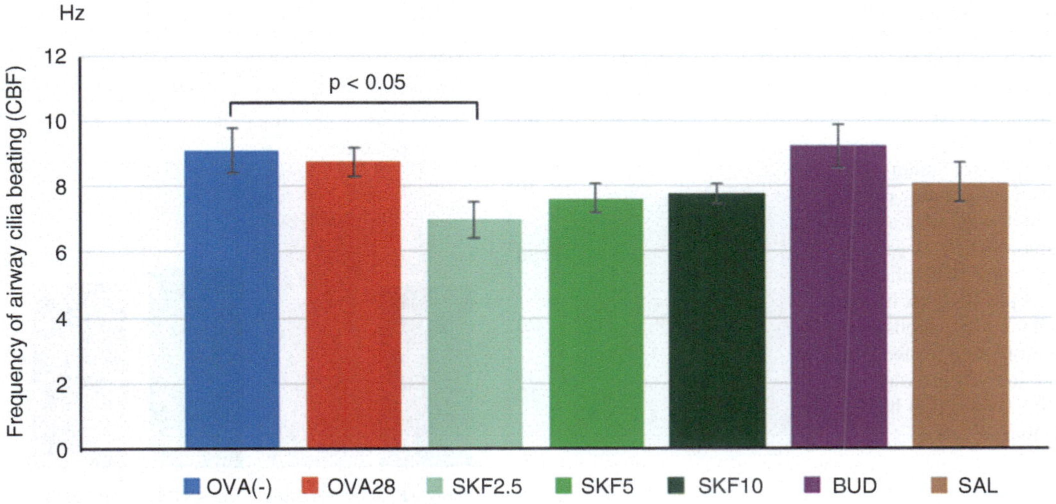

Fig. 2 Cilia beating frequency (CBF) in the investigated groups of guinea pigs: OVA(−), unsensitized control group; OVA28, ovalbumin-sensitized negative control group treated with isotonic saline; SKF2.5, 5, and 10, sensitized and treated with inhalation of SKF 96365 in the successively doubled concentrations of 2.5, 5, and 10 μM; and BUD and SAL, sensitized positive control groups treated with inhalations of budesonide and salmeterol, respectively (one-way ANOVA and post hoc Bonferroni test)

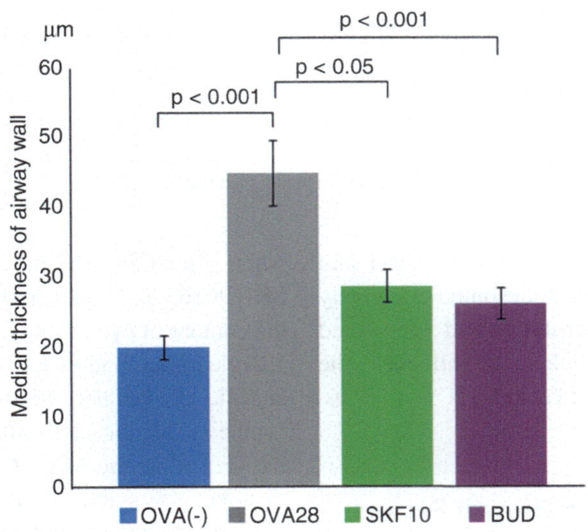

Fig. 3 Thickness of smooth muscle actin (SMA) in airway walls visualized with monoclonal SMA (1A4 clone) antibody and chromogen (3,3′-diaminobenzidine). OVA (−), unsensitized guinea pigs; OVA28, ovalbumin-sensitized negative control group treated with isotonic saline; SKF10, sensitized and treated with inhalations of 10 μM SKF 96365; and BUD, sensitized positive control group treated with budesonide (see Methods for details) (one-way ANOVA and post hoc Bonferroni test)

Specimens from the OVA(−) animals showed no signs of remodeling. Likewise, immunohistochemistry for SMA (Fig. 4) and MUC5AC showed significant expression enhancements in the sensitized negative controls (OVA28). Only was the SKF 96365 capable of reducing these AR

Fig. 4 Thickness of reticulin fibers (collagen III) in airway walls visualized with Gömöri's staining. OVA(−), unsensitized guinea pigs; OVA28, ovalbumin-sensitized negative control group treated with isotonic saline; SKF10, sensitized and treated with inhalation of 10 μM SKF 96365; and BUD, sensitized positive control group treated with budesonide (one-way ANOVA and post hoc Bonferroni test)

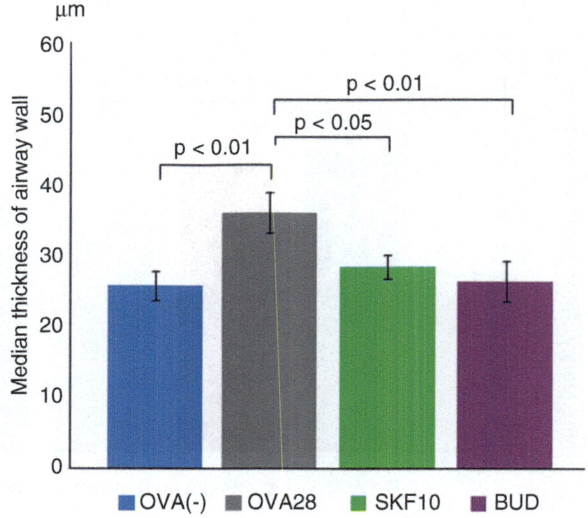

Table 1 Semi-quantitative analysis of anti-mucin 5 AC (MUC5AC) antibody positivity. The number of negative (infiltration score 0 and 1) and positive (infiltration score 2 and 3) samples in ovalbumin-unsensitized – OVA(−) guinea pigs, ovalbumin-sensitized negative controls treated with isotonic saline (OVA28), and ovalbumin-sensitized guinea pigs treated with inhalation of SKF 96365 in a concentration of 10 μM (SKF10), and ovalbumin-sensitized positive controls treated with inhalation of budesonide (BUD)

	Negative samples	Positive samples
OVA(−)	4	4
OVA28	0	10*
SKF10	5	3**
BUD	3	6

*p < 0.05 versus OVA(−); **p < 0.01 versus OVA28 (Fisher's exact test)

features, including goblet cell hyperplasia and overproduction of mucin. Budesonide effectively suppressed ASM hyperplasia and prevented fibrotic changes but failed to influence the MUC5AC enhancement (Table 1).

3.2 Cytokines and Growth Factors

Cytokine Content To gain insight into the mechanisms of AR, we quantitatively evaluated the content of key cytokines and growth factors in the lung tissue. IL-2, IL-4, IL-5, IL-10, IL-12 (p70), IL-13, TNF-α, GM-CSF, and INF-γ were examined in control OVA-sensitized untreated and treated with SKF 96365 and anti-inflammatory budesonide. IL-4, IL-5, IL-13, and IL-10 were significantly elevated in BALF collected from sensitized negative controls (OVA28) when compared to healthy unsensitized animals. SKF 96365 and budesonide significantly reduced the content of cytokines characteristic for chronic allergic inflammation and AR, such as IL-4, IL-5, and IL-13. Further, SKF 96365 enhanced the synthesis of the anti-inflammatory IL-12 and INF-γ. Unlike the SKF 96365, budesonide failed to affect the synthesis of IL-12 and INF-γ but induced a release of the anti-inflammatory IL-10. This effect, however, was significant only when compared to that in OVA(−) but not sensitized negative controls (OVA28) (Fig. 5).

Epidermal Growth Factor (EGF) and Transforming Growth Factor-Beta (TGF-β) The lung tissue EGF and TGF-β were significantly elevated after 28-day long sensitization (Fig. 6). Only SKF 96365 treatment was capable of reducing the synthesis and release of TGF-β,

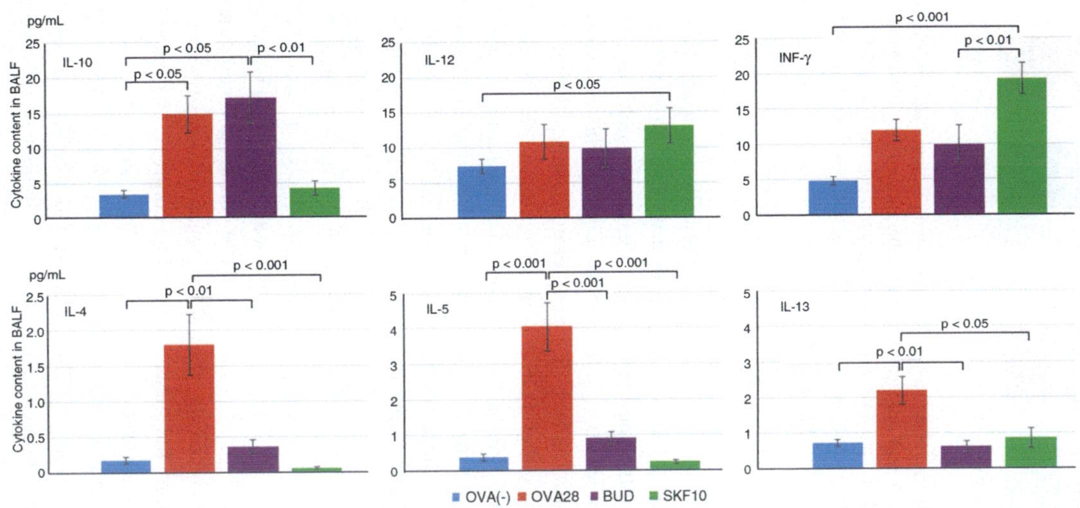

Fig. 5 Cytokine content in BALF. IL, interleukins, INF-γ, interferon-gamma; OVA (−), unsensitized guinea pigs; OVA28, ovalbumin-sensitized negative control group treated with isotonic saline; SKF10, sensitized and treated with inhalation of 10 μM SKF 96365; and BUD, sensitized positive control group treated with budesonide (one-way ANOVA and post hoc Bonferroni test)

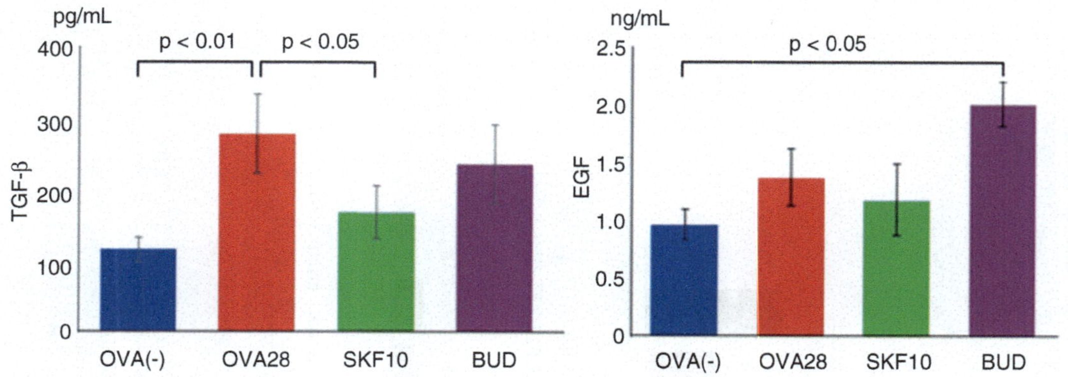

Fig. 6 Growth factors engaged in airway remodeling: transforming growth factor-beta (TGF-ß) and epidermal growth factor (EGF), evaluated in the supernatant of lung tissue homogenate. OVA(−), unsensitized guinea pigs; OVA28, ovalbumin-sensitized negative control group treated with isotonic saline; SKF10, sensitized and treated with inhalation of 10 μM SKF 96365; and BUD, sensitized positive control group treated with budesonide (one-way ANOVA and post hoc Bonferroni test)

which corresponded to an increase in IL-12 and INF-γ (BioPlex analysis), confirming the activation of the IL-12–INF-γ–TGF-β anti-remodeling pathway. However, SKF 96365 failed to significantly affect the EGF content that remained elevated. Budesonide failed to reduce either TGF-β or EGF. Since TGF-β is believed to be causally associated with goblet cells hyperplasia and mucus hyperproduction in asthma, these results are in line with the histomorphological findings outlined above.

4 Discussion

This study investigated whether blocking the CRAC channel activity could retard the airway remodeling (AR) induced on the background of chronic allergic inflammation induced by ovalbumin (OVA) sensitization in the guinea pig. The guinea pig model of allergic inflammation closely resembles the asthmatic process in the human airways. Allergen sensitization and repeated aerosolized allergen challenges are the accepted way of inducing AR, which is routinely assessed by histological examination of paraffin-embedded specimens of the airway tissue (McGovern and Mazzone 2014). Although the challenges are recommended for 12 weeks, the modified 28-day long model of chronic inflammation we used in the present study showed key AR features such as mucus hypersecretion evidenced by the enhanced MUC5AC protein expression, subepithelial fibrosis evidenced by an increase in the mass of reticulin fibers in Gömöri's staining, and ASM hyperplasia evidenced by the enhanced expression of SMA in bronchial walls. Further, we found a close association of histomorphological features of AR with the impaired airway defense mechanisms and immuno-biochemical changes, pointing to fully developed allergic inflammation, a major sign of which was a significant increase in in vivo basal and bronchoconstrictor-induced hyperreactivity-sensitized animals compared to healthy controls challenged with saline only. The CBF, a key predictor of mucociliary clearance, decreased. The AR in our model corresponded to the increased content of markers of remodeling such as the volume of elastic fibers and actin in the airway and lung tissue exposed to cumulative doses of OVA twice a week for 4 weeks (Pigati et al. 2015) or and to allergic rhinitis induced by repeated OVA intraperitoneal administration followed by intranasal challenges within 3 weeks (Chen et al. 2017) in the guinea pigs. These changes also correspond well to the epithelial airway dysfunction typical of AR in chronic asthma reported in humans where subepithelial fibrosis and mucus hypersecretion commonly result in impaired mucociliary clearance (Burgess et al. 2016; Sedaghat et al. 2016; Borish 2002; Durrani et al. 2011; Al-Muhsen et al. 2011).

In the present study, the content of IL-4, IL-5, IL-10, and IL-13 increased in BALF after 28-day long OVA sensitization in healthy guinea pigs. The IL-13, particularly, is one of the most crucial mediators of allergic inflammation. There is evidence that blocking the IL-13 in the airways alone is sufficient to prevent airway inflammation, hyperreactivity, ciliated cell loss, and mucus overproduction induced by allergen challenges in animal models of asthma (Erle and Sheppard 2014; Ford et al. 2001). IL-13-induced stimulation of the airway epithelium activates hypersecretory MUC5AC-expressing mucus cells. IL-4 appears to have effects akin to those of IL-13, as both share the common receptor on club cell, type II IL-4R whose signaling plays a role in allergen-induced mucus hyperproduction (Kuperman et al. 2005). ASM cells in asthmatic airways proliferate in response to IL-4, IL-13, and IL-5 which is a key activator of eosinophils (Halwani et al. 2010; Doherty and Broide 2007). Contrarily, the synthesis of IL-10, a prototype anti-inflammatory cytokine, decreases in asthmatic airways (Jahromi et al. 2014; Ogawa et al. 2008). Unlike the clinical condition, where the development of asthma is often associated with the immune-related predisposition, in the present experimental study we used healthy guinea pigs and repeatedly exposed them to the OVA allergen mimic allergic airway inflammation and AR. The premise was that OVA would induce chronic airway inflammatory and remodeling changes, without much immune involvement. In fact, the stimulation of protective mechanisms driven by IL-10 and IL-12 in OVA28 animals, appearing with AR, was statistically insignificant when compared to the OVA(−) group. On the other hand, 10 μM concentration of SKF 96365 not only decreased the content of the asthma-related proinflammatory cytokines production IL-4, IL-5, and IL-13 but also significantly countered the increase in the anti-inflammatory IL-12–IFN-γ pathway. The Th1 cytokines IL-12 and IFN-γ form a natural counterbalance to Th2 cytokines, driving protective cell-mediated immunity (Biedermann et al. 2004). IFN-γ secreted by Th1 cells activates macrophages and dendritic cells to produce IL-12 which, in turn, decreases the antigen-induced bronchial hyperresponsiveness, eosinophilia, and mucus goblet cell hyperplasia induced by Th2 cells (Barnes 2008; Caramori et al. 2008).

Airway structural changes are variably influenced by Th2 cytokines and growth factors. TGF-β, produced in large quantities by immune cells, fibroblasts, and epithelial cells, regulates the proliferation of immune cells and their recruitment into tissues (Bush 2019; Pakyari et al. 2013). Prochazkova et al. (2012) have shown that IL-12 is a cytokine having the ability to skew the ongoing TGF-β-dependent differentiation into Th1-like direction. IL-12 and IFN-γ production in asthmatics is often on the low side. The IL-12–INF-γ axis is considered a key downstream pathway in Th2-dependent asthma (Kim et al. 2010). Noteworthy, IL-12 activity may be countered by IL-4 action (Wong et al. 2001).

In the present study, AR features got retracted during the long-term administration of SKF 96365 in the concentration needed to selectively inhibit CRAC channels. The corticosteroid budesonide, tested in parallel for comparison, significantly inhibited ASM proliferation and increase in reticulin fiber mass but was unable to reduce mucus hypersecretion by the airway epithelium. This finding is consistent with literature data that steroids have limited effects on airway mucus hypersecretion (Shen et al. 2012). SKF 96365 exhibited similar or greater suppression of airway hyperreactivity than the classic bronchodilator salmeterol and, except for the lowest concentration tested, bronchodilatory effects were not accompanied by an adverse influence of airway cilia. Increases in the anti-inflammatory IL-12 and INF-γ caused by SKF 96365, a CRAC channel blocker, points to the possible mechanism of its anti-remodeling effect. Jia et al. (2013) have shown that mainly IL-13 enhances cytoplasmic puncta formation of ectopically expressed fluorescently tagged STIM1 and increased store-operated Ca^{2+} entry (SOCE) in ASM cells, suggesting that proinflammatory cytokines might contribute via CRAC channels to airway hyperresponsiveness. In line with this suggestion, Jairaman et al. (2016) have provided evidence that bronchial epithelial cells sense some allergens through the activation of cell surface protease-activated receptor type 2, which leads to the opening of store-operated CRAC channels. These channels are thus posed to have a central role in allergen signaling in the airway epithelium.

Corticosteroid drugs are essential anti-inflammatory drugs in the treatment of asthma. In a guinea pig asthma model of Pigati et al. (2015), dexamethasone inhibited the secretion of the pro-inflammatory Th2 cytokines IL-4, IL-5, IL-13, and TNF-α, as well as INF-γ. In this study, we used budesonide as a positive control drug and noticed the effects on cytokines in BALF akin to those exerted by dexamethasone above quoted. Moreover, budesonide tended to increase the content of IL-10, which could have a mitigating influence on AR.

The present findings also show that TGF-β and EGF increased in BALF from the OVA28 group of animals, which corresponded to histomorphological alterations. It is generally accepted that TGF-β plays a regulatory role in AR. The evidence to support the contribution of TGF-β to AR in asthma is derived from several murine and human studies (Miller et al. 2006; Flood-Page et al. 2003). TGF-β induces the apoptosis of airway epithelial cells and increases goblet cell proliferation, which suggests its role in mucus hyperproduction. TGF-β also increases fibroblast proliferation with their differentiation into myofibroblasts and the synthesis of extracellular matrix protein in subepithelial fibrosis facilitating ASM contractility and airway narrowing (Ojiaku et al. 2017; Makinde et al. 2007). Further, agonists of airway bronchoconstriction, like methacholine, enhance the release of TGF-β and other mediators from ASM cells, which augment airway narrowing and remodeling (Oenema et al. 2013; Grainge et al. 2011). Thus, TGF-β represents a bonding link for airway remodeling and hyperreactivity in asthma. The finding of the present study is that SKF 96365, inhibiting the STIM-Orai pathway, but not budesonide, significantly decreased TGF-β content in BALF. This result is in line with the study of Gao et al. (2013) where TGF-β promoted the rat ASM cell proliferation increasing STIM-Orai1 and SOCE activities, which was partially reduced by SKF-96365. While corticosteroid therapy reduces airway inflammation in asthma, the role of glucocorticoids concerning TGF-β synthesis is contentious. Some murine studies show that dexamethasone, budesonide, and fluticasone inhibit TGF-α (Takami et al. 2012) but fail to affect TGF-β (Halwani et al. 2011), while others show the anti-remodeling effect of corticosteroids mediated through a decrease in TGF-β expression (Doherty and Broide 2007; Miller et al. 2006; McMillan et al. 2005). No effects on TGF-β or inhibition of collagen deposition and mucus hyperproduction in human asthma have yet been reported (Chakir et al. 2003).

The EGF upregulates MUC5AC gene transcription by acting as a ligand for the epithelial growth factor receptor (EGFR) (Chen et al. 2016). Histamine and TNF-α act in airways by enhancing the EGFR-induced goblet cell hyperplasia (Hirota et al. 2012; Nadel 2001). The EGFR pathway ultimately activates the nuclear factor (NF)-κB, elevating the expression of genes encoding proinflammatory cytokines. The EGF also stimulates ASM hyperplasia and subepithelial fibrosis. Asthmatic airways show an increase in EGF and EGFR immunoreactivity not only in the bronchial epithelium but also in the airway glands, smooth muscles, and the thickened basement membrane (Amishima et al. 1998). Samanta et al. (2014) have shown that Ca^{2+} entry through Orai protein in human bronchial epithelial cells stimulates EGF gene expression together with c-fos and NFAT transcription factors as well as NFAT-driven gene expression. The activation of c-Fos and NFAT pathways is prevented by pre-exposure of bronchial epithelial cells to the CRAC channel blockers Synta66 and 3,5-bis-trifluoromethyl-pyrazole (BPT2). However, detectable basal EGF transcription is present in the absence of Orai-STIM pathway stimulation, which fits into the known physiological role of EGF in airway function. In the present study, neither budesonide nor SKF 96365 significantly inhibited the synthesis and release of EGF in the OVA-challenged guinea pig, the content of which was close to the level present in healthy non-sensitized animals. There is a biological plausibility that the EGFR-signaling pathway, but not EGF synthesis per se, is inhibited.

In conclusion, a 28-day-long OVA sensitization followed by inhalation challenges in the guinea pig is a valid model of asthma-like airway remodeling, in which the proinflammatory cytokines IL-4, IL-5, and IL-13, as well as TGF-ß and EGF, are involved. The structural airway alterations combined with the inflammatory process related to the magnitude of airway hyperactivity, expressed by increases in basal and constriction-induced sRaw and dysfunctional mucociliary clearance. The findings indicate that corticosteroids might have a mitigating role in remodeling, possibly through increased synthesis of IL-10. Further, we identified CRAC channels, forming an essential route of Ca^{2+} entry into airway epithelial cells, as a driving force of chronic inflammation, airway hyperactivity, and remodeling based on the reversal of the changes by the administration of a specific CRACK inhibitor, SKF 96365, in OVA-sensitized animals. The IL-12–INF-γ–TGF-β pathway activation is liable to be the underlying molecular mechanism suppressing the development of airway remodeling in response to chronic inflammation. Thus, targeting CRAC channels might offer promise as a novel therapeutic approach for managing chronic airway inflammatory disorders including advanced asthma and possibly also chronic obstructive pulmonary disease.

Acknowledgments We thank Ms. Katarina Jesenska for the outstanding technical assistance during the experimental work and Ms. Slavka Drahosova for immunohistochemical analyses. The study was supported by grants: VEGA 1/0314/21, VEGA 1/0253/19, APVV 19-0033, and the research project of the Biomedical Center Martin—ITMS 26220220187, entitled “We support research activities in Slovakia” cofinanced by the EU.

Conflicts of Interest The authors declare no conflicts of interest concerning this article.

Ethical Approval All applicable international, national, and/or institutional guidelines for the care and use of animals were followed. The animals were treated in accord with the Guide for the Care and Use of Laboratory Animals (8th edition, National Academies Press) and the EU and Slovakian legislation regulating the welfare of experimental animals. This study was approved by a local Ethics Committee of the Jessenius Faculty of Medicine in Martin, Slovakia (permit EK 40/2018), registered by the Institutional Review Board/Ethics Board Office.

References

Al-Muhsen S, Johnson JR, Hamid Q (2011) Remodelling in asthma. J Allergy Clin Immunol 128(3):451–462

Amishima M, Munakata M, Nasuhara Y, Sato A, Takahashi T, Homma Y, Kawakami Y (1998) Expression of epidermal growth factor and epidermal growth factor receptor immunoreactivity in the asthmatic human airway. Am J Respir Crit Care Med 157(6 Pt 1):1907–1912

Barnes PJ (2008) The cytokine network in asthma and chronic obstructive pulmonary disease. J Clin Invest 118(11):3546–3556

Bergeron C, Tulic MK, Hamid Q (2010) Airway remodeling in asthma: from bench side to clinical practice. Can Respir J 17(4):e85–e93

Biedermann T, Röcken M, Carballido JM (2004) Th1 and Th2 lymphocyte development and regulation of Th cell–mediated immune responses of the skin. J Invest Derm Symp Proc 9(1):5–14

Borish L (2002) The role of leukotrienes in upper and lower airway inflammation and the implications for treatment. Ann Allergy Asthma Immunol 88(4 Suppl 1):16–22

Boulet LP (2018) Airway remodeling in asthma: update on mechanisms and therapeutic approaches. Curr Opin Pulm Med 24(1):56–62

Burgess JK, Mauad T, Tjin G, Karlsson JC, Westergren-Thorsson G (2016) The extracellular matrix – the under-recognized element in lung disease? J Pathol 240(4):397–409

Bush A (2019) Cytokines and chemokines as biomarkers of future asthma. Front Pediatr 7:72

Busse P, Zhang TF, Srivastava K, Lin BP, Schofield B, Sealfon SC, Li XM (2005) Chronic exposure to TNF-α increases airway mucus gene expression *in vivo*. J Allergy Clin Immunol 116:1256–1263

Caramori G, Groneberg D, Ito K, Casolari P, Adcock IM, Papi A (2008) New drugs targeting Th2 lymphocytes in asthma. J Occup Med Toxicol 3(1):6

Chakir J, Shannon J, Molet S, Fukakusa M, Elias J, Laviolette M, Boulet LP, Hamid Q (2003) Airway remodeling-associated mediators in moderate to severe asthma: effect of steroids on TGF-beta, IL-11, IL-17, and type I and type III collagen expression. J Allergy Clin Immunol 111(6):1293–1298

Chen J, Zeng F, Forrester SJ, Eguchi S, Zhang M-Z, Harris RC (2016) Expression and function of the epidermal growth factor receptor in physiology and disease. Physiol Rev 96:1025–1069

Chen ZY, Zhou SH, Zhou QF, Tang HB (2017) Inflammation and airway remodeling of the lung in guinea pigs with allergic rhinitis. Exp Ther Med 14 (4):3485–3490

Chung SC, McDonald TV, Gardner P (1994) Inhibition by SKF 96365 of Ca^{2+}current, IL-2 production and activation in T lymphocytes. Br J Pharmacol 113 (3):861–868

Doherty T, Broide D (2007) Cytokines and growth factors in airway remodeling in asthma. Curr Opin Immunol 19(6):676–680

Durrani SR, Viswanathan RK, Busse WW (2011) What effect does asthma treatment have on airway remodeling? Current perspectives. J Allergy Clin Immunol 128(3):439–448

Erle DJ, Sheppard D (2014) The cell biology of asthma. J Cell Biol 205(5):621–631

Flood-Page P, Menzies-Gow A, Phipps S, Ying S, Wangoo A, Ludwig MS, Barnes N, Robinson D, Kay AB (2003) Anti-IL-5 treatment reduces deposition of ECM proteins in the bronchial subepithelial basement membrane of mild atopic asthmatics. J Clin Invest 112:1029–1036

Ford JG, Rennick D, Donaldson DD, Venkayya R, Hansell E, Kurup VP, Warnock M, Grünig G (2001) Il-13 and IFN-gamma: interactions in lung inflammation. J Immunol 167(3):1769–1777

Gao YD, Zheng JW, Li P, Cheng M, Yang J (2013) Store-operated Ca+ entry is involved in transforming growth factor-β1 facilitated proliferation of rat airway smooth muscle cells. J Asthma 50(5):439–448

Grainge CL, Lau LC, Ward JA, Dulay V, Lahiff G, Wilson S, Holgate S, Davies DE, Howarth PH (2011) Effect of bronchoconstriction on airway remodeling in asthma. N Engl J Med 364:2006–2015

Halwani R, Al-Muhsen S, Hamid Q (2010) Airway remodeling in asthma. Curr Opin Pharmacol 10 (3):236–245

Halwani R, Al-Muhsen S, Al-Jahdali H, Hamid Q (2011) Role of transforming growth factor-β in airway remodeling in asthma. Am J Respir Cell Mol Biol 44 (2):127–133

Hargas L, Koniar D, Stofan S (2011) In: Folea S (ed) Sophisticated biomedical tissue measurement using image analysis and virtual instrumentation, practical applications and solutions using LabVIEW™ software. IntechOpen, London. eBook (PDF) ISBN: 978-953-307-650-8; https://www.intechopen.com/books/practical-applications-and-solutions-using-labview-software. Accessed on 2 Feb 2021

Hirota N, Risse PA, Novali M, McGovern T, Al-Alwan L, McCuaig S, Proud D, Hayden P, Hamid Q, Martin JG (2012) Histamine may induce airway remodeling through release of epidermal growth factor receptor ligands from bronchial epithelial cells. FASEB J 26 (4):1704–1716

Hogan PG, Lewis RS, Rao A (2010) Molecular basis of calcium signalling in lymphocytes: STIM and ORAI. Annu Rev Immunol 28:491–533

Hostettler KE, Roth M, Burgess JK, Gencay MM, Gambazzi F, Black JL, Tamm M, Borger P (2008) Airway epithelium-derived transforming growth factor-beta is a regulator of fibroblast proliferation in both fibrotic and normal subjects. Clin Exp Allergy 38 (8):1309–1317

Jahromi SR, Mahesh PA, Jayaraj BS, Madhunapantula SRV, Holla AD, Vishweswaraiah S, Ramachandra NB (2014) Serum levels of IL-10, IL-17F and IL-33 in patients with asthma: a case-control study. J Asthma 51(10):1004–1013

Jairaman A, Maguire CH, Schleimer RP, Prakriya M (2016) Allergens stimulate store-operated calcium entry and cytokine production in airway epithelial cells. Sci Rep 6:32311

Jia L, Delmotte P, Aravamudan B, Pabelick CM, Prakash YS, Sieck GC (2013) Effects of the inflammatory cytokines TNF-α and IL-13 on stromal interaction molecule-1 aggregation in human airway smooth muscle intracellular Ca^{2+} regulation. Am J Respir Cell Mol Biol 49(4):601–608

Kim YS, Choi SJ, Choi JP, Jeon SG, Oh S, Lee BJ, Gho YS, Lee CG, Zhu Z, Elias JA, Kim YK (2010) IL-12-STAT4-IFN-gamma axis is a key downstream pathway in the development of IL-13-mediated asthma phenotypes in a Th2 type asthma model. Exp Mol Med 42(8):533–546

Kuperman DA, Huang X, Nguyenvu L, Hölscher C, Brombacher F, Erle DJ (2005) IL-4 receptor signaling in Clara cells is required for allergen-induced mucus production. J Immunol 175(6):3746–3752

Mahn K, Ojo OO, Chadwick G, Aaronson PI, Ward JP, Lee TH (2010) Ca^{2+} homeostasis and structural and functional remodeling of airway smooth muscle in asthma. Thorax 65(6):547–552

Makinde T, Murphy RF, Agrawal DK (2007) The regulatory role of TGF-beta in airway remodeling in asthma. Immunol Cell Biol 85(5):348–356

McGovern AE, Mazzone SB (2014) Guinea pig models of asthma. Curr Protoc Pharmacol 67: Unit:5.26.1–5.26.38

McMillan SJ, Xanthou G, Lloyd C (2005) Therapeutic administration of budesonide ameliorates allergen-induced airway remodeling. Clin Exp Allergy 35 (3):388–396

Miller M, Cho JY, McElwain K, McElwain S, Shim JW, Manni M, Baek JS, Broide DH (2006) Corticosteroids prevent myofibroblast accumulation and airway remodeling in mice. Am J Physiol Lung Cell Mol Physiol 290(1):162–169

Munakata M (2006) Airway remodelling and airway smooth muscle in asthma. Allergol Int 55:235–243

Nadel JA (2001) Role of epidermal growth factor receptor activation in regulating mucin synthesis. Respir Res 2 (2):85–89

Oenema TA, Maarsingh H, Smit M, Groothuis GMM, Meurs H, Gosens R (2013) Bronchoconstriction induces TGF-b release and airway remodeling in guinea pig lung slices. PLoS One 8(6):e65580

Ogawa Y, Duru EA, Ameredes BT (2008) Role of IL-10 in the resolution of airway inflammation. Curr Mol Med 8 (5):437–445

Ojiaku CA, Yoo EJ, Panettieri RA (2017) Transforming growth factor β1 function in airway remodelling and hyperresponsiveness. The missing link? Am J Respir Cell Mol 56(4):432–442

Pakyari M, Farrokhi A, Maharlooei MH, Ghahary A (2013) Critical role of transforming growth factor beta in different phases of wound healing. Adv Wound Care 2(5):215–224

Pennock BE, Cox CP, Rogers RM, Cain WA, Wells JH (1979) A noninvasive technique for measurement of changes in specific airway resistance. J Appl Physiol 46:399–406

Perez-Zoghbi JF, Karner C, Ito S, Shepherd M, Alrashdan Y, Sanderson MJ (2009) Ion channel regulation of intracellular calcium and airway smooth muscle function. Pulm Pharmacol Ther 22(5):388–397

Pigati PA, Righetti RF, Possa SS, Romanholo BS, Rodrigues AP, dos Santos AS, Xisto DG, Antunes MA, Prado CM, Leick EA, Martins Mde A, Rocco PR, Tibério Ide F (2015) Y-27632 is associated with corticosteroid-potentiated control of pulmonary remodeling and inflammation in guinea pigs with chronic allergic inflammation. BMC Pulm Med 15:85

Prochazkova J, Pokorna K, Holan V (2012) IL-12 inhibits the TGF-β-dependent T cell developmental programs and skews the TGF-β-induced differentiation into a Th1-like direction. Immunobiology 217(1):74–82

Samanta K, Parekh AB (2016) Store-operated Ca^{2+} channels in airway epithelial cell function and implications for asthma. Philos Trans R Soc Lond Ser B Biol Sci 371(1700):20150424

Samanta K, Bakowski D, Parekh AB (2014) Key role for store-operated Ca^{2+} channels in activating gene expression in human airway bronchial epithelial cells. PLoS One 9(8):e105586

Sedaghat MH, Shahmardan MM, Norouzi M, Heydari M (2016) Effect of cilia beat frequency on muco-ciliary clearance. J Biomed Phys Eng 6(4):265–278

Shen Y, Chen L, Wang T, Wen F (2012) PPARγ as a potential target to treat airway mucus hypersecretion in chronic airway inflammatory diseases. PPAR Res 2012:256874

Shore S (2002) Airway smooth muscle: new tricks for an old dog. Am J Physiol Lung Cell Mol Physiol 282(3): L518–L519

Singh A, Hildebrand ME, Garcia E, Snutch TP (2010) The transient receptor potential channel antagonist SKF 96365 is a potent blocker of low-voltage-activated T-type calcium channels. Br J Pharmacol 160 (6):1464–1475

Spinelli AM, Trebak M (2016) Orai channel-mediated Ca^{2+} signals in vascular and airway smooth muscle. Am J Physiol Cell Physiol 310(6):C402–C413

Spinelli AM, González-Cobos JC, Zhang X, Motiani RK, Rowan S, Zhang W, Garrett J, Vincent PA, Matrougui K, Singer HA, Trebak M (2012) Airway smooth muscle STIM1 and Orai1 are upregulated in asthmatic mice and mediate PDGF-activated SOCE, CRAC currents, proliferation, and migration. Pflugers Arch 464(5):481–492

Sutovska M, Kocmalova M, Joskova M, Adamkov M, Franova S (2015) The effect of long-term administered CRAC channels blocker on the functions of respiratory epithelium in guinea pig allergic asthma model. Gen Physiol Biophys 34(2):167–176

Sutovska M, Kocmalova M, Franova S, Vakkalanka S, Viswanadha S (2016) Pharmacodynamic evaluation of RP3128, a novel and potent CRAC channel inhibitor in guinea pig models of allergic asthma. Eur J Pharmacol 772:62–70

Takami S, Mizuno T, Oyanagi T, Tadaki H, Suzuki T, Muramatsu K, Takizawa T, Arakawa H (2012) Glucocorticoids inhibit MUC5AC production induced by transforming growth factor-α in human respiratory cells. Allergol Int 61(3):451–459

Vig M, DeHaven WI, Bird GS, Billingsley JM, Wang H, Rao PE, Hutchings AB, Jouvin MH, Putney JW, Kinet JP (2008) Defective mast cell effector functions in mice lacking the CRACM1 pore subunit of store-operated calcium release-activated calcium channels. Nat Immunol 9(1):89–96

Wong CK, Ho CY, Ko FWS, Chan CHS, Ho ASS, Hui DSC, Lam CWK (2001) Proinflammatory cytokines (IL-17, IL-6, IL-18 and IL-12) and Th cytokines (IFN-γ, IL-4, IL-10 and IL-13) in patients with allergic asthma. Clin Exp Immunol 125(2):177–183

Adv Exp Med Biol - Clinical and Experimental Biomedicine (2022) 13: 103–109
https://doi.org/10.1007/5584_2020_610

Published online: 31 December 2020

In Silico Analysis of Bone Tension During Fixation of the Medial Malleolus Fracture After Ankle Joint Endoprosthesis

Jacek Lorkowski, Renata Wilk, and Mieczysław Pokorski

Abstract

Total ankle arthroplasty (TAR) is a procedure alternative to arthrodesis which enables the biomechanical stabilization of the ankle joint. The procedure is associated with a high risk of complications, including fractures of the medial malleolus. In this study, the finite element method (FEM), based on CT examinations, was used to model the ankle fracture fixation after TAR. Three types of fracture stabilization were considered: screw, Blount staple, and both screw and Blount staple. In the *in silico* model, the maximum stress tension was found at prosthetic junctions with the base, cone, and talar components of the tibial prosthesis. When the fracture was stabilized with the Blount staple, tension along the cone of the tibial component was about 12% of the maximum tension. Stabilizations with the screw alone or Blount staple combined with a screw on the medial side of the cone induced tension in the immediate vicinity twice as high. In the area of the medial malleolus, the tension was alike for both types of stabilization. The tension was lowest when using the Blount staple alone. We conclude that, contrary to the hitherto clinical routine of using screws, fracture fixation using the Blount staple leads to the lowest bone tension around the fixation of the medial malleolus fracture after ankle joint endoprosthesis.

Keywords

Ankle arthroplasty · Ankle joint · *In silico* · Finite elements · Periprosthetic fracture · Talocrural joint

1 Introduction

Total ankle arthroplasty (TAR) is a procedure more and more frequently performed. Contrary to the hip and knee joints arthroplasty, the reason for its implementation is usually not primary, but secondary to post-traumatic degenerative changes. The TAR is an alternative to arthrodesis that disrupts the proper functioning of the articular chain in the lower limb and impairs the entire

J. Lorkowski (✉)
Department of Orthopedics and Traumatology, Central Clinical Hospital of Ministry of Interior, Warsaw, Poland

Faculty of Health Sciences, Medical University of Mazovia, Warsaw, Poland
e-mail: jacek.lorkowski@gmail.com

R. Wilk
Department of Anatomy, Faculty of Health Science in Katowice, Medical University of Silesia, Katowice, Katowice, Poland
e-mail: renatawilk@poczta.onet.pl

M. Pokorski
Institute of Health Sciences, Opole University, Opole, Poland

Faculty of Health Sciences, The Jan Długosz University in Częstochowa, Częstochowa, Poland
e-mail: m_pokorski@hotmail.com

biomechanics of the locomotor system (Morash et al. 2017; Basques et al. 2016). The currently used third-generation ankle prostheses provide better biomechanical fit and survival of endoprostheses than the previous generations, although it is not the only factor determining survival (Zafar et al. 2020). Among many factors qualifying and disqualifying to the TAR, particular attention is paid to the lack of vascular impairments in the operated limb. From the biomechanical standpoint and to avoid perioperative complications, good bone stock is a key factor (Van der Plaat and Haverkamp 2017).

Ankle arthroplasty procedures, although provide better biomechanical results when compared to arthrodesis, show a significantly higher percentage of complications that mostly depend on the learning curve that describes the progress in the surgeon's experience in performing the procedure (Morash et al. 2017; Basques et al. 2016). One of the complications often arising during the implantation of an ankle joint endoprosthesis is a periprosthetic fracture. At present, the number of intraoperative fractures is decreasing but postoperative fractures are on the rise (Haendlmayer et al. 2009). The most common fractures occurring during endoprosthesis implantation concern the medial or lateral malleolus. They usually result from the use of oscillating saws and accidental cuts of the ankle or from oversizing the endoprosthesis. The reported incidence of periprosthetic fractures varies among studies. Manegold et al. (2013) have reported the incidence of 2.2%, whereas Lee et al. (2013) put the incidence of medial malleolus fractures at 10% and lateral malleolus fractures at 0.6%. In a study by Clough et al. (2018), intraoperative medial fractures accounted for 9.7% of all ankle arthroplasty procedures performed. Zaidi et al. (2013) have also reported that medial malleolus fractures as the commonest complication of arthroplasty, with an incidence of 6% compared to 1% for the lateral malleolus. It appears that as the number of procedures increases, the incidence of intraoperative fractures declines (Basques et al. 2016). Nevertheless, the issue of periprosthetic fractures in the case of TAR remains clinically significant as it affects up to 10% of patients, which makes it essential to search for the optimal method of fracture stabilization.

The finite element method (FEM) is increasingly used to define the biomechanics of fracture stabilization (Jiang et al. 2019; Anwar et al. 2017). The method enables prompt computer-based modeling and visualization of biomechanical tensions at the ankle periprosthetic fracture (Lorkowski et al. 2015, 2020). The present study aimed to create an *in silico* model of tensions arising in the medial malleolus and endoprosthesis itself using different types of fracture stabilization. Such modeling could help clarify the unresolved issue of which type of stabilization in use carries the lowest risk of implant destabilization and failure of the entire ankle arthroplasty.

2 Methods

We developed an *in silico* model of the ankle joint after arthroplasty, specifically targeted at a fracture of the medial ankle. The model was based on three clinical cases. The modeled prosthesis was of the third generation, consisting of a tibial component with a cone, a talar component made of metal alloys, and a polyethylene insert. The evaluation of bone tension arising at the bone-endoprosthesis interface transversely passing through the medial malleolus was compared between the following methods of periprosthetic fracture stabilization:

- Cortical screw passing through the medial malleolus from its apex to the shaft of the tibia, transversely through the fracture gap
- Blount staple inserted with its tines above and below the fracture gap in the medial malleolus, stabilizing the fracture externally on the medial surface of the malleolus
- Combination of these two types of stabilization, i.e., a cortical screw and Blount staple.

The bone tension, arising after fracture stabilization, was compared to that generated at the bone-endoprosthesis interface without fracture. For modeling, we used computer tomography

(CT) images of the ankle joint of an exemplary patient with an implanted joint endoprosthesis. The images, presented as a bitmap in 256 shades of gray, were processed using the software-based image registration technique to quantify tension-induced metabolic bone changes on CT images, which enables the assigning of material features to each shade of gray in the image. The resultant tension displacements at the bone-implant interface were then elaborated using the FEM 2D modeling in the ANSYS software (Ansys Inc. 2010), which enables the evaluation of tension appearing in the mechanics of solids under the influence of various factors. The area FEM-tested is divided into simple finite elements with specific geometric shapes (triangles) connected by several points at the edges, forming "knots". After selecting the nodal functions that determine the distribution of the tested physical quantity within the finite elements, calculations in the differential equations enable the determination of knots' behavior while for other points they remain approximate. After introducing the boundary conditions for the system of equations used, it is possible to determine the type and degree of displacement in nodes, which reflects tension changes present in individual parts of the bone-implant system and fracture stabilization elements (Lorkowski et al. 2020).

Based on the X-ray images, a 2D model of the ankle joint tissues and the implanted prosthesis was prepared. Overall, 16 components were obtained visible on the contour map. The images show the components representing a particular type of tissue-like bones, articular cartilage, soft elements, parts of the endoprosthesis, and elements used to fracture stabilization (Fig. 1). Young's modulus, equal to the longitudinal stress divided by the strain, and Poisson's ratio, described as a ratio of the transverse strain in the direction perpendicular to the applied force and axial strain in the direction of the applied force, were calculated for individual tissues and stabilization elements (Table 1). The former is a measure of elasticity or the ability of a bone to resist changes in length when under longitudinal tension and the latter is the ability of a bone to expand in the direction perpendicular to the direction of compression. The transverse fracture gap in the medial malleolus was modeled and then, computer models of various types of fracture stabilization were made. The models included the fracture stabilization with a screw passing through the fracture gap along the long axis of

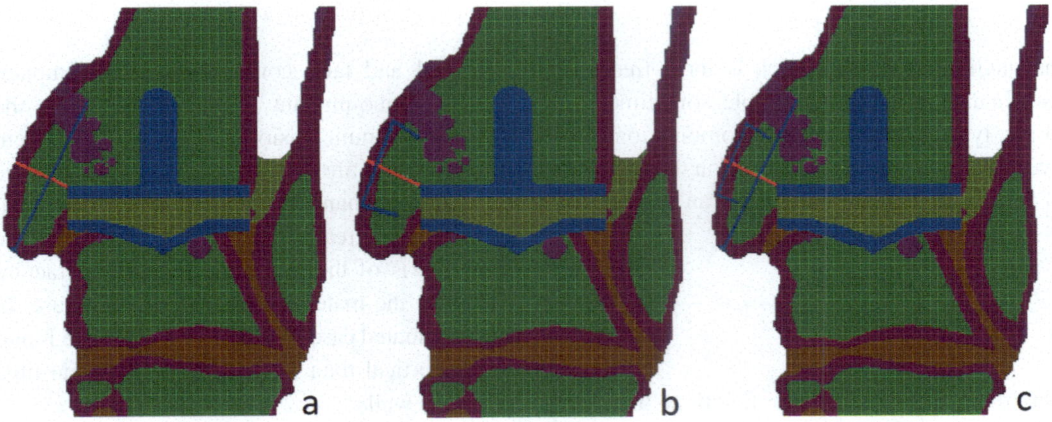

Fig. 1 A 2D ankle tissue model with implanted endoprosthesis and the stabilization elements of the medial malleolus fracture. Fracture gap marked by a red stroke on the left-hand side: (**a**) cortical screw passing through the malleolus from its apex to the shaft of the tibia, transversely through the fracture gap; (**b**) Blount staple inserted with its tines above and below the fracture gap in the medial malleolus, stabilizing the fracture externally on the medial surface of the malleolus; (**c**) combination of the cortical screw and Blount staple

Table 1 Young's modulus and Poisson's coefficient of individual tissues and elements of endoprostheses used for ankle fracture stabilization

Material	Young's modulus	Poisson's coefficient
Bone	5000 MPa	0.32
Cartilage	150 MPa	0.42
Soft tissues	800 MPa	0.42
Implant	210 GPa	0.32
Stabilization components	210 GPa	0.32

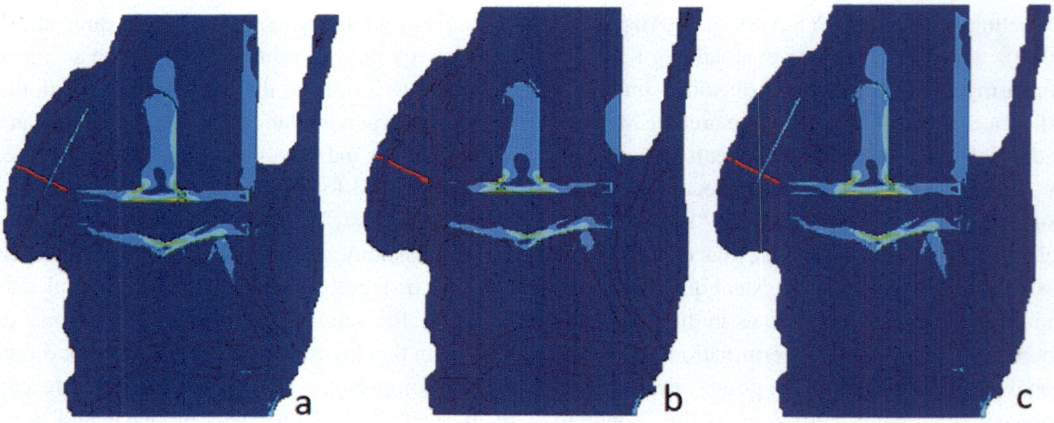

Fig. 2 Bone tension evaluation (stress distribution) arising at the bone-endoprosthesis area after total ankle arthroplasty and stabilization of the medial malleolus fracture. Fracture gap marked by a red stroke on the left-hand side: (**a**) cortical screw passing through the medial malleolus from its apex to the shaft of the tibia, transversely through the fracture gap; (**b**) Blount staple inserted with its tines above and below the fracture gap in the medial malleolus, stabilizing the fracture externally on the medial surface of the malleolus; (**c**) combination of the cortical screw and Blount staple

the medial malleolus, which is most frequently used in the clinic, a Blount staple, sometimes used in this type of fracture, and a combination of the two. The FEM model was based on the force load of $F_\lambda = 7.28$ N, determined from an average load of 1 N/1 mm^3.

3 Results

Maximum tensions locally found at the bone-implant interface in the *in silico* model was 8.4 MPa. This magnitude of tension was found without a fracture or healed fracture at the base of the medial malleolus. Similar tensions were noted in the malleolus fracture fixed with a screw alone, Blount staple, and a Blount staple and screw together. Tensions arose in the central parts of the tibial and talar components of the implant and the bone-implant interface. However, the area of maximum tension in the tibial component covered the entire cone base and was about three times larger than that in the talar component (Fig. 2). The greatest tension occurred along the central axis of the limb, and not in the fracture fissure or the material stabilizing the fracture. In each evaluated case, greater overloads were found in the cortical than medial layers of lateral tibia and talus walls.

When the fracture gap was stabilized with the Blount staple alone (Fig. 2b), tension along the cone of the tibial component was about 12% of the maximum tension. The use of a screw alone or together with the Blount staple (Fig. 2a, c) doubled up the tension on the medial side of the cone of the tibial component and about the immediate vicinity. Additionally, stabilizing elements exert tension forces of similar magnitude in the extension of the tibia cone, targeting the posterior tibia wall. In the area of the medial malleolus, tensions were alike when stabilizing the fracture with a screw or together with the Blount staple. Tensions arising in the joining materials reached one-third of the maximum tension occurring in the entire biomechanical system in the case of screw alone or together with the Blount staple and one-fourth of the maximum tension in the case of Blount staple alone.

4 Discussion

In this study, we used a rapid FEM computer-driven modeling to evaluate tensions arising at the bone, endoprosthesis, and bone-endoprosthesis interface after total ankle arthroplasty. The modeling seems particularly useful in the assessment and prevention of the potential propensity for a fracture of the medial malleolus, an adverse event stemming from arthroplasty. The method is based on CT scans of the leg bones with an implanted ankle joint endoprosthesis, transformed into 2D images, aimed at providing the prompt evaluation results intraoperatively. The distribution of tensions arising after the endoprosthetic-related medial malleolus fracture was evaluated with the content of a stabilizing central cone in the tibial component. Noteworthy, we found differences in the magnitude and localization of tension depending on the way of fracture gap stabilization. In detail, the tension along the prosthetic cone of the tibial component approximated 12% of the maximum stress using the Blount staple. Stabilization with the Blount staple and screw together or a screw alone induced tensions on the medial side of the tibial cone component and its immediate vicinity twice as much.

According to the classification of Manegold et al. (2013), malleolus fractures are stratified into Type 1 – intraoperative fractures, type 2 – postoperative fractures resulting from a fall, and type 3 – fractures resulting from both bones overload and physiological stress on deficient elastic resistance. Concerning the exact location of a fracture site, the classification distinguishes type A – medial malleolus, type B – lateral malleolus, C – tibia, and D – talus. Fractures have the essential bearing on the implant stability, so an additional stratification distinguishes stable from unstable implants, anonymized as S and U, respectively, based on the X-ray or CT examination. Our present finite element model fits well into type 1AU intraoperative fractures. However, the model would also be adequate for those type 2 fractures in which there are no significant changes in bone anatomy apart from the fracture gap. Type 3 fractures are usually linked to altered bone structure. Therefore, the model would barely reflect clinical reality.

The prevalence of periprosthetic fractures arising during surgery can be as high as 20% (Brock et al. 2017; Manegold et al. 2013). In periprosthetic ankle fractures, it is recommended to use surgical stabilization to prevent displacement in the case of both intra- and postoperative fractures (Cody et al. 2018). The conservative treatment is recommended only for non-displaced fractures of the medial malleolus. Nonetheless, even in such fractures, the non-union occurs in 12–13% (Tsitsilonis et al. 2015). Intraoperative periprosthetic fractures are most often stabilized using Kirschner wires (K-wires), screws (Barnes et al. 2014), or locking plates (LCP) (Jiang et al. 2019). In some cases, Blount staples are used with satisfactory results (Schiedts et al. 1997). These methods have been studied in many aspects, but no consensus has been reached as to which one is the most effective. The prevalence of non-union in medial malleolus fractures ranges from 3% to 20% (Corey et al. 2019), which may result in implant destabilization. Jiang et al. (2019) have used the FEM for the evaluation of different types of stabilization in medial malleolus fractures and found that a screw inserted along the long axis of the medial malleolus from its apex, when the fracture gap runs horizontally, did not provide good results. Mounting a screw was not sufficient to prevent displacement. Further, tensions arising below the screw could chip the bone away and, as a result, the screw may go loose or fall out, causing severe pain as the screw head is close under the skin. The use of headless compression screws mitigates this problem in the stabilization of medial malleolus fractures and reduces the percentage of non-unions. The perception of pain after endoprosthesis stabilization exceeds *in silico* analysis. The suboptimal nature of prosthetic stabilization using screws alone is consistent with our present results.

The locking plates are another way to stabilize malleolar fractures, which was subject to finite element analysis (Anwar et al. 2017). The plates prevent bone damage and the fallout of a screw by transferring a portion of the tension from the screw placed along with the locking plate to the shaft of the tibia. Unfortunately, there is a danger of breaking a locking plate. Besides, mounting the plates using screws is technically difficult and not always feasible due to a restricted intraoperative area. The current stabilization systems of prosthetic fractures of the medial malleolus still fall short of the requirements of effectiveness. The search continues for new methods that would provide better effectiveness and safety of the obtained fracture unions.

Blount staples have been used for years in epiphysiodesis, i.e., correcting discrepancies in limb length in children or for correcting valgus knees (genu valgum) or claw knees (genu varum), showing as good results as other corrective modalities, e.g., the eight-plate method (Rodrigues et al. 2020). In the treatment of medial malleolus fractures, the use of Blount staples is not common, but a study by Schiedts et al. (1997) has shown promising results. A new technique of Blount staples placement developed by Burghardt et al. (2012) requires a smaller skin incision and provides easier access to the bone and a stable union of the fracture, which raises interest in using it in a greater number of orthopedic procedures in both children and adults. Patients whose fractures are a consequence of the implantation of an ankle joint endoprosthesis may benefit from this method as well. Therefore, in the present study, we used the finite element method to model the stabilization of the medial malleolus fracture after ankle arthroplasty using Blount staples. We demonstrate a lower level of tensions developing in the endoprosthesis area, which carries a lower risk of endoprosthesis destabilization and procedure failure, and therefore a lower risk of reoperation and arthrodesis. This study has limitations inherent for the theoretical analysis that requires assumptions about the patient's condition, bone quality, and the type of fracture we are dealing with. Nonetheless, we believe we have shown that, contrary to the hitherto clinical routine of using screws, fracture fixation using the Blount staple leads to a lower bone tension about the stabilization of the medial malleolus fracture after ankle joint endoprosthesis. The assessment of a potential practical reference of the proposed fixation method as well as perioperative finite element modeling requires alternative clinically oriented study designs.

Conflicts of Interest The authors declare no competing interests in relation to this article.

Ethical Approval All procedures performed in this study involving human medical data complied with the ethical standards of the institutional and/or national research committee and with the 1964 Helsinki declaration and its later amendments or comparable ethical standards. This article concerned computer modeling based on anonymous clinical data. As it contains no identifiable personal data, no patient consent was required.

References

ANSYS Inc (2010) Release 13 documentation for ANSYS

Anwar A, Lv D, Zhao Z, Zhang Z, Lu M, Nazir MU, Qasim W (2017) Finite element analysis of the three different posterior malleolus fixation strategies in relation to different fracture sizes. Injury 48:825–832

Barnes H, Cannada LK, Watson JT (2014) A clinical evaluation of alternative fixation techniques for medial malleolus fractures. Injury 45(9):1365–1367

Basques BA, Bitterman A, Campbell KJ, Haughom BD, Lin J, Lee S (2016) Influence of surgeon volume on inpatient complications, cost and length of stay following total ankle arthroplasty. Foot Ankle Int 37 (10):1046–1051

Brock AK, Tan EW, Shafiq B (2017) Post-traumatic periprosthetic tibial and fibular fracture after total ankle arthroplasty: a case report. J Foot Ankle Surg 56:196–200

Burghardt RD, Kanellopoulos AD, Herzenberg JE (2012) A technical note on improved instrumentation for Blount staple insertion. J Child Orthop 6:347–350

Clough TM, Alvi F, Majeed H (2018) Total ankle arthroplasty: what are the risks: a guide to surgical consent and a review of the literature. Bone Joint J 100-B(10):1352–1358

Cody EA, Scott DJ, Easley ME (2018) Total ankle arthroplasty: a critical analysis review. JBJS Rev 6(8):8e

Corey RM, Cannada LK, Bledsoe G, Israel H (2019) Biomechanical evaluation of medial malleolus fractures treated with headless compression screws. J Clin Orthop Trauma 10(2):310–314

Haendlmayer KT, Fazly FM, Harris NJ (2009) Periprosthetic fracture after total ankle replacement: surgical technique. Foot Ankle Int 3(12):1233–1234

Jiang D, Zhan S, Wang Q, Ling M, Hu H, Jia W (2019) biomechanical comparison of locking plate and cancellous screw techniques in medial malleolar fractures: a finite element analysis. J Foot Ankle Surg 58:1138–1144

Lee KT, Young KW, Kim JB, Seo YS (2013) Perioperative complications and learning curve of the mobility total Ankle System. Foot Ankle Int 34:210–214

Lorkowski J, Mrzygłód MW, Grzegorowska O, Kotela I (2015) An *in silico* analysis of ankle joints loads in secondary ankle osteoarthritis. Case study. Ortop Traumatol Rehabil 17(3):305–315

Lorkowski J, Wilk R, Pokorski M (2020) *In silico* evaluation of treatment of periprosthetic fractures in elderly patients after hip arthroplasty. Adv Exp Med Biol. https://doi.org/10.1007/5584_2020_555. Epub ahead of print. PMID: 32567038

Manegold S, Haas NP, Tsitsilonis S, Springer A, Märdian S, Schaser KD (2013) Periprosthetic fractures in total ankle replacement: classification system and treatment algorithm. J Bone Joint Surg Am 95 (9):815–820. S1-3

Morash J, Walton DM, Glazebrook M (2017) Ankle arthrodesis versus total ankle arthroplasty. Foot Ankle Clin N Am 22:251–266

Rodrigues NVM, Guarniero R, Villas Boas PJF, Miranda BR, Montenegro NB (2020) Hemiepiphysiodesis using eight-plate *versus* Blount staple to correct genu valgum and genu varum. Acta Ortop Bras 28(4):195–198

Schiedts D, Fleurat E, Bouger D, Bastaraud H (1997) Osteosynthesis of internal malleolar fracture by staplers. Rev Chir Orthop Reparatrice Appar Mot 83 (1):70–73

Tsitsilonis S, Schaser KD, Wichlas F, Haas NP, Manegold S (2015) Functional and radiological outcome of periprosthetic fractures of the ankle. Bone Joint J 97-B:950–956

Van der Plaat LW, Haverkamp D (2017) Patient selection for total ankle arthroplasty. Orthop Res Rev 9:63–73

Zafar MJ, Kallemose T, Benyahia M, Ebskov LB, Ostergaard Penny J (2020) 12-years survival analysis of 322 Hintegra total ankle arthroplasties from an independent center. Acta Orthop 91(4):444–449

Zaidi R, Cro S, Gurusamy K, Sivanadarajah N, Macgregor A, Henricson A, Goldberg A (2013) The outcome of total ankle replacement. A systematic review and meta-analysis. Bone Joint J 95-B:1500–1507

Adv Exp Med Biol - Clinical and Experimental Biomedicine (2022) 13: 111–119
https://doi.org/10.1007/5584_2021_627

Published online: 20 March 2021

Effects of Physical Activity at High Altitude on Hormonal Profiles in Foreign Trekkers and Indigenous Nepalese Porters

Alessandro Tafuri, Danilo Bondi, Alessandro Princiotta, Tiziana Pietrangelo, Pabitra Yadav, Vincenzo Maria Altieri, Maria Angela Cerruto, Fiore Pelliccione, Alessandro Antonelli, and Vittore Verratti

Abstract

Altitude exposure affects hormonal homeostasis, but the adaptation of different populations is still not finely defined. This study aims to compare the mid-term effects of combining physical activity and altitude hypoxia on hormonal profiles in foreign trekkers coming from Italy versus indigenous Nepalese porters during a Himalayan trek. Participants (6 Italians and 6 Nepalese) completed a 300 km distance in 19 days of an accumulated altitude difference of 16,000 m, with an average daily walk of 6 h. The effect of high altitude on hormonal pathways was assessed by collecting blood samples the day before the expedition and the day after its completion. Foreign trekkers had an additional follow-up sample collected after 10 days. The findings revealed a different

A. Tafuri
Department of Neuroscience, Imaging and Clinical Sciences, University "G. d'Annunzio" of Chieti – Pescara, Chieti, Italy

Department of Urology, University of Verona, Azienda Ospedaliera Universitaria Integrata Verona, Verona, Italy
e-mail: aletaf@hotmail.it

D. Bondi and T. Pietrangelo
Department of Neuroscience, Imaging and Clinical Sciences, University "G. d'Annunzio" of Chieti – Pescara, Chieti, Italy
e-mail: danilo.bondi@unich.it; tiziana.pietrangelo@unich.it

A. Princiotta, M. A. Cerruto, and A. Antonelli
Department of Urology, University of Verona, Azienda Ospedaliera Universitaria Integrata Verona, Verona, Italy
e-mail: alessandroprinciotta0@gmail.com; mariaangela.cerruto@univr.it; alessandro_antonelli@me.com

P. Yadav
Clinical Biochemistry Unit, Bir Hospital, Kathmandu, Nepal
e-mail: yadavpabitra8@gmail.com

V. M. Altieri
U.O. Urologia, Policlinico di Monza, Monza, Italy
e-mail: vincenzomaria.altieri@gmail.com

F. Pelliccione
Department of Internal Medicine, Diabetes and Metabolism Unit, Azienda ASL 02 Chieti - Lanciano - Vasto, F. Renzetti Hospital, Lanciano, Italy
e-mail: fiore.pelliccione@gmail.com

V. Verratti (✉)
Department of Psychological, Health and Territorial Sciences, University "G. d'Annunzio" of Chieti – Pescara, Chieti, Italy
e-mail: vittore.verratti@unich.it

adaptation of thyroidal and gonadal axes to mid-term strenuous physical activity combined with high-altitude hypobaric hypoxia. The thyroid function shifted to the protective mechanism of low free triiodothyronine (FT3), whereas the gonadal axis was suppressed. The Italian trekkers and Nepalese porters had lower total testosterone and 17-β-estradiol levels after the expedition. At the follow-up, the Italians had increased testosterone values. Prolactin secretion decreased in the Italians but increased in the Nepalese. We conclude that exposure to high-altitude affects the hormonal axes. The effect seems notably pronounced for the hypothalamus-pituitary gonadal axis, suppressed after high-altitude exposure.

Keywords

Foreign trekkers · High altitude · Hormonal axis · Hypobaric hypoxia · Nepalese porters · Physical activity

1 Introduction

From the pioneering work of Hans Selye on endocrinology and adaptation syndrome, the hypothalamic-pituitary axis has been recognized as the main player in the homeostatic adaptation to psychological or physical stressors (Rochette and Vergely 2017). Among the environmental stressors, high altitude has been steadily growing in interest during the last decades, considering the spread of altitude traveling. High altitude affects human systems impacting their physiological activities due to hypobaric hypoxia and climatic condition. It has been shown that central and peripheral endocrine functions are affected by high altitude, usually above 5000 m, barring persistent human colonization (von Wolff et al. 2018). The high-altitude hypoxic model is usually adopted to study the pathophysiologic effects of low oxygen tension in the aging process or cardiorespiratory disorders (Verratti et al. 2016; Cataldi and Di Giulio, 2009). Chronic conditions can also impair hormonal metabolism affecting target organs' activities. However, findings in various studies are highly contentious, which may be caused by the wide diversity in the length and degree of hypoxic exposure, gender, age, and environmental conditions (Keenan et al. 2019; Verratti et al. 2017; Park et al. 2014).

Humans of different ethnicity, exposed from birth to different levels of hypoxia, respond and adapt to acute and chronic high-altitude exposure in diverse ways (Magliulo et al. 2020; Verratti et al. 2021). Comparisons of changes in hormonal profiles between different ethnicities, including sojourners and natives, in relation to high altitude are scarce. Researchers have focused on highland dwellers, trekkers, or climbers, somehow leaving out a population of altitude porters who have a specific geographic origin and often suffer from high altitude illness (Dawadi et al. 2020). The motivation behind the study of porters also lies in their legendary performance during uphill loaded locomotion, playing a fundamental role in the success of altitude expeditions (Minetti et al. 2006), as opposed to altitude travelers for whom the physical strain involved limits the performance and poses substantial stress. In this study, we address the effects of altitude hypoxia on hormonal profiles in foreign trekkers versus indigenous Nepalese porters during an altitude trek in the Himalayas.

2 Methods

2.1 Participants and Study Protocol

This study was conducted in accord with the STAR Data Reporting Guidelines for Clinical High Altitude Research (Brodmann Maeder et al. 2018). Six Italian trekkers and six indigenous native Nepalese porters took part in the trial, which was a separate ramification of the research project "Kanchenjunga Exploration & Physiology". The basic demographics of the participants are presented in Table 1. Participants completed a 300 km distance in 19 days of an accumulated altitude difference of 16,000 m, with an average daily walk of 6 h. The route involved demanding ascents and descents in the Kanchenjunga region in the Himalayas in Nepal (Fig. 1). The

Table 1 Participants' characteristics – The Himalayan "Kanchenjunga Exploration & Physiology" expedition

Ethnicity	Gender	Age (year)	BMI pre (kg/m^2)	BMI post (kg/m^2)
Caucasian (Italians)	Female	36	25.07	24.65
	Male	63	28.91	27.34
	Male	59	21.91	21.35
	Male	25	24.31	23.13
	Male	32	24.14	23.14
	Male	48	30.54	27.98
Mean ± SD		44 ± 15	25.8 ± 3.3	24.6 ± 2.6
Indo-Aryan (Nepalese)	Male	26	26.49	25.66
	Male	18	17.51	16.88
	Male	39	22.99	22.38
	Male	40	28.83	27.77
	Male	30	29.41	28.38
	Male	29	20.94	21.34
Mean ± SD		30 ± 8	24.4 ± 4.7	23.7 ± 4.4

BMI Body mass index, a day before and a day after the expedition

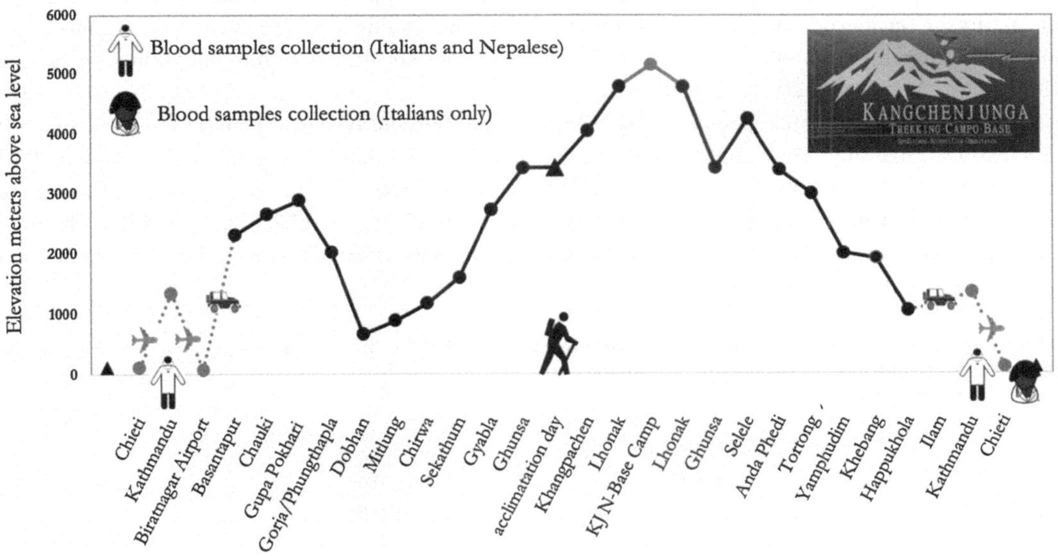

Fig. 1 Altimetric plan of "Kanchenjunga Exploration & Physiology" expedition

expedition was supervised by a trained doctor who monitored symptoms, peripheral blood oxygen saturation (SpO_2), arterial blood pressure, and anthropometric data throughout the whole period. None of the participants suffered acute mountain sickness.

Blood samples were collected from the antecubital vein, stored in vacutainer serum tubes, and immediately centrifuged at 3000 rpm × 10 min in the Bir Hospital (Kathmandu, Nepal, 1340 m), the day before and the day after the Himalayan trek. The serum was stored frozen at −5 °C and transported to Italy for later analyses in the Laboratory of Clinical Pathology of Teramo Hospital in the city of Teramo. Additionally, Italian participants' serum was collected and analyzed at a 10-day follow-up once they returned to Italy.

The blood content of hormones was determined using the immuno-chemiluminescence assay in the ADVIA Centaur XP Immunoassay System (Siemens Healthcare; Erlangen Germany). We assayed thyroid function – free triiodothyronine (FT3), free thyroxine (FT4), thyroid-stimulating hormone (TSH), the hypothalamus-pituitary-gonadal axis – total testosterone, follicle-stimulating hormone (FSH), luteinizing hormone (LH), estradiol, and the prolactin cortisol pathways.

2.2 Statistical Analysis

Normality of data distribution was assessed with the Shapiro-Wilk, the equality of variances with the Levene test, and whether the two data sets came from populations with a common distribution was determined with the quantile-quantile (Q-Q) plots. Considering the presence of missing points, we run a mixed-model analysis for all the parameters (Armstrong 2017). Specifically, we used the general linear mixed model (GLMM), with restricted maximum likelihood (REML) estimation and likelihood ratio testing (LRT) for random effects, time × ethnicity comparisons, and participants as the random variable. In the case of foreign participants, this analysis concerned pre vs. post vs. follow-up comparisons. The post hoc tests were conducted with the Bonferroni correction for multiple comparisons. The Satterthwaite method for degrees of freedom was used, and partial eta squared (η^2_p) and partial omega squared (ω^2_p) were calculated as measures of effect size (Fritz et al. 2012). The analysis was performed using R-based open-source Jamovi v1.2.5.0 software (https://www.jamovi.org).

3 Results

3.1 Thyroid Function

Thyroid-Stimulating Hormone Changes in TSH in both Italian and Nepalese participants after altitude exposure were unremarkable (Table 2).

Free Triiodothyronine (FT3) The investigation of thyroid function showed a reduction in FT3 concentration from pre-to-post altitude exposure ($p = 0.012$, $\eta^2_p = 0.525$, $\omega^2_p = 0.448$). The time × ethnicity comparison revealed a tendency for a

Table 2 Hormonal blood serum content in the Italian trekkers and Nepalese porters during exposure to high altitude in Kanchenjunga Exploration & Physiology" expedition

	Pre	Post	Follow-up
	TSH (μg/mL)		
Italians	1.26 ± 0.66	1.20 ± 0.64	1.08 ± 0.73
Nepalese	1.73 ± 0.81	1.61 ± 0.58	–
	FSH (mUI/mL)		
Italians	5.11 ± 1.48	4.96 ± 1.00	5.07 ± 0.96
Nepalese	5.84 ± 2.00	5.05 ± 2.36	–
	LH (mUI/mL)		
Italians	2.73 ± 1.00	3.26 ± 1.05	3.33 ± 0.55
Nepalese	4.26 ± 2.42	4.60 ± 1.61	–
	Cortisol (μ g/mL)		
Italians	9.41 ± 2.52	10.30 ± 2.73	10.81 ± 3.78
Nepalese	9.59 ± 3.79	8.59 ± 2.41	–

TSH Thyroid-stimulating hormone, *FSH* Follicle-stimulating hormone, *LH* Luteinizing hormone. Measurements were done a day before (pre) and a day after (post) the trek in the blood serum. An additional measurement was done at a 10-day follow-up in the Italians only. Changes in the serum content of hormones depicted in the table both between pre/post altitude exposure and between the ethnicities failed to reach statistical significance

difference ($p = 0.078$, $\eta^2_p = 0.306$, $\omega^2_p = 0.212$), with the Italian participants showing a greater reduction (from 2.75 ± 0.15 to 2.20 ± 0.46 pg/mL; $p = 0.016$) than the Nepalese (from 2.76 ± 0.31 to 2.63 ± 0.23 pg/mL) in post hoc analysis. At a 10-day follow up, FT3 reverted to the baseline level in the Italians (2.87 ± 0.35 pg/mL), as revealed by the pre vs. post vs. follow-up comparison ($p = 0.011$, $\eta^2_p = 0.703$, $\omega^2_p = 0.599$), and significant post hoc differences were found (pre vs. post: $p = 0.037$ and post vs. follow-up: $p = 0.020$). The random effect of participants was not significant, and the effect sizes for the overall model were as follows: R^2 marginal = 0.352, R^2 conditional = 0.569.

Free Thyroxine (FT4) In the Italian participants, FT4 content increased from pre-to-post altitude exposure, the increase persisted at a 10-day follow-up (1.07 ± 0.20 pg/mL, 1.21 ± 0.08 pg/mL, and 1.20 ± 0.09 pg/mL, respectively). In the Nepalese, we found an opposite trend, with FT4 reduction after altitude exposure (1.27 ± 0.14 pg/mL and 1.15 ± 0.08 pg/mL, respectively). Moreover, time × ethnicity comparison revealed a significant difference ($p = 0.025$, $\eta^2_p = 0.443$, $\omega^2_p = 0.359$). The random effect of participants was not significant, and the effect sizes for the overall model were as follows: R^2 marginal = 0.248, R^2 conditional = 0.425.

3.2 Hypothalamus-Pituitary-Gonadal and Hypothalamus-Pituitary-Adrenal Axes

Gonadotropins Changes in FSH and LH in both Italian and Nepalese participants after altitude exposure were unremarkable (Table 2).

Testosterone The content of total testosterone decreased from pre-to-post altitude exposure, albeit the changes were of borderline significance ($p = 0.109$, $\eta^2_p = 0.260$, $\omega^2_p = 0.164$), with the Nepalese participants having a greater reduction (from 4.56 ± 0.82 ng/mL to 3.40 ± 1.30 ng/mL) when compared with the Italians (from 4.86 ± 1.68 ng/mL to 4.35 ± 0.95 ng/mL); the difference between the two ethnic groups was insignificant (Fig. 2). At a 10-day follow up in the Italian participants, the baseline testosterone significantly increased to 6.57 ± 1.38 ng/mL, as revealed by the pre vs. post vs. follow-up comparison ($p = 0.038$, $\eta^2_p = 0.675$, $\omega^2_p = 0.515$), and post-hoc differences were found (pre vs. post: $p = 0.161$ and post vs. follow-up: $p = 0.043$). The random effect of participants was not significant, and the effect sizes for the overall model were as follows: R^2 marginal = 0.181, R^2 conditional = 0.335.

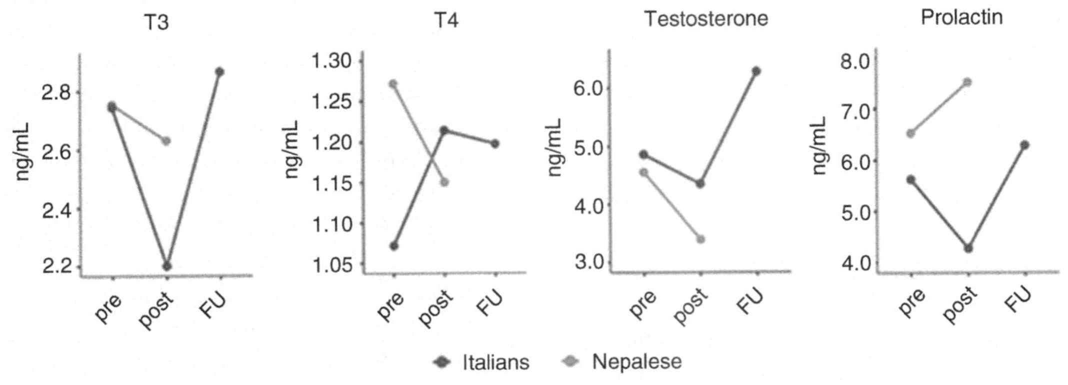

Fig. 2 Hormonal adaptations during exposure to high altitude in the Italian trekkers and Nepalese porters in Kanchenjunga Exploration & Physiology" expedition. Measurements were done a day before (pre) and a day after (post) the trek in the blood serum. An additional measurement was done at a 10-day follow-up (FU) in Italians only

17-β-Estradiol In the Italian participants, 17-β-estradiol content decreased from the pre-altitude exposure level of 30.98 ± 3.20 pg/mL to 11.80 pg/mL post-exposure, which was the lower detection limit, and reverted at a 10-day follow-up to 30.52 ± 2.73 pg/mL. In the Nepalese, a reduction in 17-β-estradiol after exposure was variably expressed; three of them had a massive decrease from 19.60 ± 3.36 pg/mL to below the detection limit of 11.80 pg/mL, another two had a modest decrease, on average, from 24.05 pg/mL to 21.68 pg/mL, and it tended to increase in one subject from 11.80 pg/mL to 12.80 pg/mL.

Stress Hormones Changes in cortisol in both Italian and Nepalese participants after altitude exposure were unremarkable (Table 2).

Considering prolactin, it decreased from pre-to-post altitude exposure in the Italian participants to bounce back, exceeding the baseline level at a 10-day follow-up (5.63 ± 1.39 ng/mL, 4.28 ± 1.34 ng/mL, and 6.11 ± 0.19 ng/mL, respectively), as revealed by the pre vs. post vs. follow-up comparison ($p = 0.009$, $\eta^2_p = 0.741$, $\omega^2_p = 0.642$), and post-hoc differences were found (pre vs. post: $p = 0.068$ and post vs. follow-up: $p = 0.010$). Contrarily, in the Nepalese, prolactin increased from pre-to-post exposure (6.53 ± 2.38 ng/mL and 7.52 ± 2.22 ng/mL, respectively); time × ethnicity comparison revealed a borderline difference ($p = 0.148$, $\eta^2_p = 0.218$, $\omega^2_p = 0.120$). The random effect of participants was not significant, and the effect sizes for the overall model were as follows: R^2 marginal = 0.281, R^2 conditional = 0.432.

4 Discussion

High altitude affects human systems influencing their physiological activities due to hypobaric hypoxia and climatic environment. Hypoxia per se influences oxidative metabolism, stimulating compensatory mechanisms to ensure proper oxygenation of tissues (Di Giulio et al. 2006). Central and peripheral endocrine functions, such as hormonal pathways, are affected by altitude above 5000 m, preventing persistent human colonization (von Wolff et al. 2018). In the present chapter, we investigated whether a combination of physical effort and hypobaric hypoxia was associated with a perturbation of hormonal profile in a group of foreign trekkers coming from Italy when compared with indigenous Nepalese porters.

The thyroidal axis showed an adaptive mechanism characterized by a reduction in the serum level of FT3 both in foreign and Nepalese trekkers. The FT4 level showed ethnically reversing features, increasing in the foreigners and decreasing in the Nepalese. The TSH level remained unchanged. The FT3 and FT4 levels reverted to the baseline pre-altitude exposure value in the foreign trekkers at a 10-day follow-up. Richalet et al. (2010) have reported a 16% increase in both total and free T3 after 3–4 days of stay at 4350 m. Contrarily, we found a reduction in T3 after the altitude trek, which was more accentuated in the foreign trekkers than the Nepalese porters. A reduction in T3 is typical of non-thyroidal illness syndrome (NTIS), which occurs in various stressful non-thyroidal illnesses and during starvation. Under such conditions, peripheral conversion of T4 to T3 is reduced in the presence of normal thyroid hormone secretion resulting in an FT3 decrease, while FT4 may be unchanged, decreased, or increased. The NTIS is underlain by impaired conversion of T4 to T3 due to enzymatic dysfunction of deiodinases. The low-T3 syndrome caused by reduced peripheral conversion of the prohormone T4 is also present in chronic inflammatory diseases. As a result, inflammation disrupts redox homeostasis, inhibiting the hypothalamic-pituitary-thyroid axis. Hypothyroidism that follows exacerbates the redox homeostasis disruption, further worsening the activity of deiodinase. Our findings suggest that a reduction in T3 might involve the same inflammatory redox pathway that drives the low-T3 syndrome (Mancini et al. 2016). Further, there is a biological plausibility that indigenous porters in Nepal have an innate protective mechanism sparing the function of deiodinases.

We found in this study that the gonadal hormone axis was partially suppressed as confirmed by a non-significant reduction in testosterone levels and a significant decrease in 17-β-estradiol after the expedition in both foreign and Nepalese participants. These findings are in line with those of Benso et al. (2007), who found reductions in serum testosterone in eight mountaineers at the base camp located at 5200 m during a Mount Everest expedition. Marinelli et al. (1994) have reported a prompt decrease in serum testosterone occurring within 24 h after exposure to high altitude. Thus, the possibility arises that an inappreciable reduction in testosterone we observed after days of trekking during the expedition could be due to a delayed blood sampling which enabled the rebound of testosterone level, likely triggered by increased LH. Hypobaric hypoxia, rather than physical effort, seems the main reason for a transient reduction in testosterone as prolonged strenuous physical activity in endurance athletes or marathon runners at sea level fails to show appreciable effects on circulating reproductive hormones (Lucía et al. 1996; Jensen et al. 1995; Bagatell and Bremner 1990). Noteworthy, we found a significant increase in serum testosterone in foreign trekkers at follow-up, the finding in line with a previous study in which testosterone increased 10 days after the end of prolonged trekking at 5900 m in seven male mountaineers, which could be related to changes in the body composition (Pelliccione et al. 2011).

We also found that serum prolactin decreased in the Italian trekkers at high altitude with a reversal to the baseline level at the 10-day follow-up. It is a reasonable assumption that altitude hypoxia mitigates the activation of lactotroph cells in the anterior pituitary resulting in less prolactin secretion, which may be a sign of general bodily suffering of foreign sojourners at altitude. Likewise, Benso et al. (2007) have found a significant increase in serum prolactin in Caucasian mountaineers after climbing Mount Everest. The authors suggest changes in prolactin reciprocate those in testosterone. Somewhat in line with this suggestion, we found that prolactin increased from the pre-to-post trek in the Nepalese porters, a reverse reflection of those in testosterone. The ingenious high-altitude settlers perform physically better compared to foreigners even though they usually are exposed to a greater physical load.

The present study also shows that serum cortisol was not appreciably affected by high-altitude trekking. The lack of effect of cortisol content is in line with the findings of Wolff et al. (2018), who have conducted a major study on cerebral, cardiovascular, pulmonary, and humoral adaptations to prolonged hypobaric hypoxia during an ascent to Mt. Himlung Himal (7126 m) in Nepal, involving forty healthy sojourners, 21 men and 19 women aged 18–70. In that study, serum cortisol was slightly modulated with increasing altitude, changes were unrelated to sex or arterial oxygen saturation, and the level of cortisol after the expedition was akin to that before it. That study, in line with our present findings, also shows that prolactin secretion and thyroid function are affected by increasing altitude and the gonadal hormonal axis is suppressed, with reversal of changes to the baseline levels at a follow-up.

In conclusion, we believe we have shown that brain-driven humoral responses are modulated by a prolonged strenuous effort during a Himalayan high-altitude trek. The accompanying hypobaric hypoxia appeared to notably affect the hypothalamus-pituitary gonadal axis suppressing serum testosterone and 17-β-estradiol contents; the effects were more pronounced in indigenous Nepalese porters than in foreign Caucasian sojourners. Hypobaric hypoxia also shifted the thyroid metabolic function to the protective way of low free triiodothyronine level, the effect was more pronounced in Caucasian sojourners. There is a degree of ethnic diversity in specific humoral changes toward the stronger adaptive downregulation of humoral function in high-altitude native Nepalese. This adaptation may underlie their superior performance in the physically loaded condition, when compared to foreign sojourners, due possibly to the ensuing lower cellular ATP demand mitigating the effects of oxygen depletion at high altitude. Generally, however, the ethnic differences in humoral responses were modest and reversible on return from the trek in both Caucasians and native Nepalese. The exact molecular mechanisms of humoral changes underlying the effects of high-altitude hypobaric hypoxia could not be resolved in this observational study. Further research, particularly considering the diurnal response, in addition to sequential assessments during altitude exposure, is needed to provide insights into ethnicity-dependent differential responses to physical effort at high altitude.

Acknowledgments Supported by a grant from the Department of Psychological, Health and Territorial Sciences of "G. d'Annunzio" University of Chieti-Pescara, Italy. Our thanks for the logistic support go to the Mission Nepal Holidays Pvt. Ltd. in Kathmandu, Nepal, the Laboratory of Clinical Pathology of Teramo Hospital, the Clinical Biochemistry Unit in the Bir Hospital in Kathmandu, and the Unique Diagnostic Polyclinic Laboratory in Kathmandu. We also thank all participating trekkers.

Competing Interests The authors declare no competing interests in relation to this chapter.

Ethical Approval All procedures performed in studies involving human participants were in accord with the ethical standards of the institutional and/or national research committee and with the 1964 Helsinki declaration and its later amendments or comparable ethical standards. This project was approved by the Ethics Review Board of the Nepal Health Research Council (NHRC).

Informed Consent Written informed consent was obtained from all individual participants included in the study.

References

Armstrong RA (2017) Recommendations for analysis of repeated-measures designs: testing and correcting for sphericity and use of MANOVA and mixed model analysis. Ophthalmic Physiol Opt 37(5):585–593

Bagatell CJ, Bremner WJ (1990) Sperm counts and reproductive hormones in male marathoners and lean controls. Fertil Steril 53(4):688–692

Benso A, Broglio F, Aimaretti G, Lucatello B, Lanfranco F, Ghigo E, Grottoli S (2007) Endocrine and metabolic responses to extreme altitude and physical exercise in climbers. Eur J Endocrinol 157(6):733–740

Brodmann Maeder M, Brugger H, Pun M, Strapazzon G, Dal Cappello T, Maggiorini M, Hackett P, Bärtsch P, Swenson ER, Zafren K (2018) The STAR data reporting guidelines for clinical high altitude research. High Alt Med Biol 19(1):7–14

Cataldi A, Di Giulio C (2009) Oxygen supply as modulator of aging processes: hypoxia and hyperoxia models for aging studies. Curr Aging Sci 2(2):95–102

Dawadi S, Basnyat B, Adhikari S (2020) A review of medical problems in Himalayan porters. High Alt Med Biol 21(2):109–113

Di Giulio C, Bianchi G, Cacchio M, Artese L, Piccirilli M, Verratti V, Valerio R, Iturriaga R (2006) Neuroglobin, a new oxygen binding protein is present in the carotid body and increases after chronic intermittent hypoxia. Adv Exp Med Biol 580:15–19

Fritz CO, Morris PE, Richler JJ (2012) Effect size estimates: current use, calculations, and interpretation. J Exp Psychol Gen 141(1):2–18

Jensen CE, Wiswedel K, McLoughlin J, van der Spuy Z (1995) Prospective study of hormonal and semen profiles in marathon runners. Fertil Steril 64(6):1189–1196

Keenan DM, Pichler Hefti J, Veldhuis JD, Von Wolff M (2019) Regulation and adaptation of endocrine axes at high altitude. Am J Physiol Endocrinol Metab 318(2): E297–E309

Lucía A, Chicharro JL, Pérez M, Serratosa L, Bandrés F, Legido JC (1996) Reproductive function in male endurance athletes: sperm analysis and hormonal profile. J Appl Physiol 81(6):2627–2636

Magliulo L, Bondi D, Pietrangelo T, Fulle S, Piccinelli R, Jandova T, Blasio GD, Taraborrelli M, Verratti V (2020) Serum ferritin and vitamin D evaluation in response to high altitude comparing Italians trekkers vs Nepalese porters. Eur J Sport Sci:1–9. https://doi.org/10.1080/17461391.2020.1792559

Mancini A, Di Segni C, Raimondo S, Olivieri G, Silvestrini A, Meucci E, Currò D (2016) Thyroid hormones, oxidative stress, and inflammation. Mediat Inflamm 2016:6757154

Marinelli M, Roi GS, Giacometti M, Bonini P, Banfi G (1994) Cortisol, testosterone, and free testosterone in athletes performing a marathon at 4,000 m altitude. Horm Res 41(5–6):225–229

Minetti AE, Formenti F, Ardigò LP (2006) Himalayan porter's specialization: metabolic power, economy, efficiency and skill. Proc Biol Sci 273 (1602):2791–2797

Park JY, Hwang TK, Park HK, Ahn RS (2014) Differences in cardiovascular and hypothalamic-pituitary-adrenal axis functions between high altitude visitors and natives during a trek on the Annapurna circuit. Neuroendocrinology 99(2):130–138

Pelliccione F, Verratti V, D'Angeli A, Micillo A, Doria C, Pezzella A, Iacutone G, Francavilla F, Di Giulio C, Francavilla S (2011) Physical exercise at high altitude is associated with a testicular dysfunction leading to reduced sperm concentration but healthy sperm quality. Fertil Steril 96(1):28–33

Richalet JP, Letournel M, Souberbielle JC (2010) Effects of high altitude hypoxia on the hormonal response to hypothalamic factors. Am J Physiol Regul Integr Comp Physiol 299(6):R1685–R1692

Rochette L, Vergely C (2017) Hans Selye and the stress response: 80 years after his "letter" to the Editor of Nature. Ann Cardiol Angéiologie 66(4):181–183

Verratti V, Di Giulio C, D'Angeli A, Tafuri A, Francavilla S, Pelliccione F (2016) Sperm forward motility is negatively affected by short-term exposure to altitude hypoxia. Andrologia 48(7):800–806

Verratti V, Ietta F, Paulesu L, Romagnoli R, Ceccarelli I, Doria C, Fanò Illic G, Di Giulio C, Aloisi AM (2017) Physiological effects of high altitude trekking on gonadal, thyroid hormones and macrophage migration inhibitory factor (MIF) responses in young lowlander women. Physiol Rep 5(20):e13400

Verratti V, Bondi D, Shakir A, Pietrangelo T, Piccinelli R, Altieri VM, Migliorelli D, Tafuri A (2021) Uroflowmetry and altitude hypoxia: a report from healthy Italian trekkers and Nepalese porters during Himalayan expedition. Adv Exp Med Biol 1289:99–105

von Wolff M, Nakas CT, Tobler M, Merz TM, Hilty MP, Veldhuis JD, Huber AR, Pichler Hefti J (2018) Adrenal, thyroid and gonadal axes are affected at high altitude. Endocr Connect 7(10):1081–1089

Adv Exp Med Biol - Clinical and Experimental Biomedicine (2022) 13: 121–127
https://doi.org/10.1007/5584_2021_628

Published online: 14 March 2021

Influence of Parathyroidectomy on Sleep Quality in Primary Hyperparathyroidism

Renan Viola Rasche, Frauke Schuster, Natalie Meurer, Theodora Margariti, Norbert Weyerbrock, Kurt Rasche, and Cornelia Dotzenrath

Abstract

We investigated the impact of parathyroidectomy on sleep quality in patients with primary hyperparathyroidism (pHPT). Thirty consecutive patients with pHPT were enrolled in the study within 1 year. pHPT was diagnosed by typical symptoms accompanied by an elevated level of parathormone. The Pittsburgh Sleep Quality Index (PSQI) was used for the evaluation of sleep 1 day before and 6 months after parathyroidectomy. The mean total PSQI score was elevated to 6.8 ± 0.6 points before surgery, which was in the pathological cut-off of greater than ≥ 5, indicating impaired sleep quality. After parathyroidectomy, the total score declined insignificantly, amounting to 5.6 ± 0.4 ($p > 0.05$). Nevertheless, the number of patients with a score of ≥ 5 before surgery decreased from 21 (70%) to 16 (53%) after surgery. There also was a significant improvement in sleep latency ($p = 0.05$) and sleep efficiency ($p = 0.02$) domains of PSQI. We conclude that 70% of patients with untreated pHPT suffered from sleep disorders that improved after parathyroidectomy. The clinical consequence is that patients with pHPT should be questioned about having sleep disorders, which might influence the decision-making concerning parathyroidectomy. With the relation reversed, patients without pHPT but suffering from sleep disturbance should be tested for pHPT.

Keywords

Hyperparathyroidism · Parathyroidectomy · Sleep disorders · Sleep quality

R. V. Rasche, F. Schuster, N. Meurer, T. Margariti, N. Weyerbrock, and C. Dotzenrath (✉)
Department of Endocrine Surgery, Helios University Hospital Wuppertal, University of Witten-Herdecke and Heinrich-Heine University Düsseldorf, Wuppertal, Germany
e-mail: renan-rasche@hotmail.de; fschuster@yahoo.de; natalie.meurer@helios-gesundheit.de; Dorothymarg@gmail.com; norbert.weyerbrock@helios-gesundheit.de; cornelia.dotzenrath@helios-gesundheit.de

K. Rasche
Department of Pneumology, Allergology, Sleep and Respiratory Medicine, Helios University Hospital Wuppertal, University of Witten-Herdecke, Heusnerstr, Wuppertal, Germany
e-mail: kurt.rasche@helios-gesundheit.de

1 Introduction

Primary hyperparathyroidism (pHPT) is caused by adenomas of the parathyroid gland. This benign disease is characterized by parathyroid hyperfunction. Serum parathormone and calcium levels are elevated. A definite therapy can only be achieved by parathyroidectomy

(Miedlich et al. 2002). Classical symptoms and comorbidities of pHPT are kidney stones, bone diseases, and neuromuscular dysfunction. Patients also suffer from other unspecific symptoms like weakness, fatigue, depression, anxiety, irritability, cognitive dysfunction, and sleep disturbance (Liu et al. 2020; Pasieka et al. 2009; Mittendorf et al. 2007; Weber et al. 2007; Dotzenrath et al. 2006; Lundgren et al. 1998). This study aims to investigate the influence of parathyroidectomy on sleep quality in patients with pHPT.

2 Methods

2.1 Patients and Protocol

A total of 30 consecutive patients with pHPT were enrolled in the study for 1 year. There were 26 women and 4 men in the study, aged 57 ± 2 years, with the body mass index (BMI) of 26.3 ± 0.9 kg/m^2. The pHPT was diagnosed due to the presence of typical symptoms and the elevated serum levels of parathormone and calcium. All patients underwent a parathyroidectomy. The sleep quality was evaluated 1 day before and 6 months after surgery using the Pittsburgh Sleep Quality Index (PSQI). Exclusion criteria were a PSQI score of ≤ 3 according to the classification of the American Society of Anesthesiologists (ASA), secondary HPT, and the inability to understand the German language. There were no dropouts.

2.2 Pittsburgh Sleep Quality Index (PSQI)

The PSQI is a validated questionnaire that assesses subjective sleep quality during the last 4 weeks. The survey contains 18 items in 7 domains. Aside from general sleep quality, it assesses sleep latency, efficiency, duration, sleep-disturbing events, the use of sleep medication, daytime sleepiness, and fatigue (DGSM 2007a, b). The domains are scored from 0 to 2. These values sum up for the total score ranging from 0 to 21. The higher the total score, the worse is the sleep quality. When the total score is ≥ 5, the patient is assumed to suffer from sleep disturbance (Buysee et al. 1989).

Data were expressed as mean $\pm$ SD. Intergroup differences were tested using Student's *t*-test for independent samples or by a χ^2-test in case of non-normal distribution. A p-value <0.05 defined statistically significant differences. The analysis was done using MS Excel for Windows.

3 Results

3.1 Patients

The serum PTH and Ca^{2+} before parathyroidectomy were increased to 211.7 ± 135.3 ng/L and 2.8 ± 0.2 mmol/L, respectively. Six months after the operation, both declined to the normal range of 34.9 ± 14.4 ng/L and 2.3 ± 0.1 mmol/L, respectively. Patients had several typical pHPT comorbidities before parathyroidectomy, such as osteoporosis – 3 (10%) patients, a fracture of a lumbar vertebra – 1 (3%), kidney stones – 4 (12%), and gastrointestinal disorders – 7 (23%).

3.2 Pittsburgh Sleep Quality Index (PSQI) Score

The mean value of the total PSQI score was 6.8 ± 0.6 before parathyroidectomy. This score was in the pathological range of ≥ 5 in 21 out of the 30 (70%) patients, indicating impaired sleep quality. After surgery, the score tended to decline, amounting to 5.6 ± 0.4. It remained elevated above 5 points in 16 (53%) patients. The mean pre/postoperation difference of 1.2 ± 0.1 was insignificant. The evaluation of specific PSQI domains yielded variable results.

Sleep Quality Before parathyroidectomy, 16 patients had "very good" or "quite good" subjective sleep quality and 14 patients "quite bad" or "very bad" sleep quality. After the operation, 20 patients had "very good" or "quite good" sleep quality and 10 patients had "quite bad" or "very bad" sleep quality. The tendency for the amelioration of sleep disturbance after surgery failed to reach statistical significance ($p = 0.29$).

Sleep Latency Before parathyroidectomy, 21 patients scored 0 or 1 (0 = sleep latency <30 min, 1 = sleep latency >30 min less than once in a week), 9 patients scored 2 or 3 (2 = sleep latency >30 min two or three times a week, 3 = sleep latency >30 min more than three times a week). After surgery, 27 patients scored 0 or 1 and 3 patients scored 2 or 3, which led to a significant reduction in sleep latency ($p = 0.05$).

Sleep Duration Before parathyroidectomy, 19 patients slept for six or more hours *per* night. After surgery, the number of such patients increased to 24. Although this difference failed to reach statistical significance, there was a consistent impression that parathyroidectomy tended to extend sleep duration.

Sleep Efficiency Sleep efficiency is defined as the percentage of time spent asleep while in bed (DGSM 2007a). A normal level of sleep efficiency is set at 85% or higher. Before parathyroidectomy, 11 patients had sleep efficiency greater than 85%. After surgery, 20 patients reached this level of sleep efficiency; the effect was significant ($p = 0.02$).

Sleep Disorders Concerning sleep disorders, patients had to answer the question of how often *per* week and for what reason they wake up at night. Before parathyroidectomy, 20 patients reported up to 2 awakenings *per* week, which was considered normal, and 10 patients had more than 2 awakenings *per* week. Surgery failed to appreciably change the number of nightly awakenings, with 19 and 11 patients, respectively ($p = 0.79$).

Sleep Medications Patients had to answer the question how often they used sleep medications in the past 4 weeks, prescribed or acquired over the counter. Before parathyroidectomy, 27 patients reported taking sleep medications less than once a week compared to 28 patients after the operation. The remaining patients were taking sleep medications once a week or more often. Thus, the surgery failed to influence the necessity to use sleep medications ($p = 0.64$).

Daytime Sleepiness The assessment of daytime sleepiness consisted of two questions. The first question concerned the potential problems with staying awake during car driving, eating, or social encounters and the other concerned the problems with handling daily chores in the past 4 weeks. Twenty-two patients before parathyroidectomy and 26 after it did not report the increased daytime sleepiness, as opposed to 8 and 4 patients, respectively, who did report an increase in sleepiness. There was no significant pre/postsurgery change in daytime sleepiness ($p = 0.20$). The PSQI assessment data above outlined are summarized in Fig. 1.

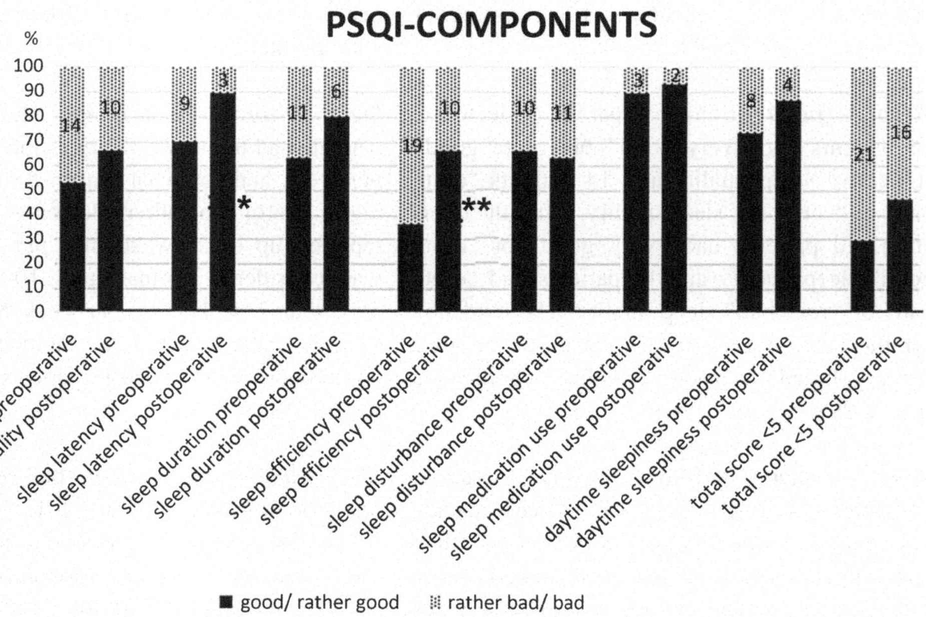

Fig. 1 Percentage and the absolute number of patients with primary hyperparathyroidism with good/rather good (black) versus bad/rather bad (dotted) scores in Pittsburgh Sleep Quality Index (PSQI) pre/post parathyroidectomy. Total number of patients in each vertical bar was 20; $^{*}p = 0.05$; $^{**}p = 0.02$

4 Discussion

Several studies of the last years have investigated cognitive and neuro-psychological changes, sleep quality, and the quality of life in patients with pHPT (Kearns et al. 2019; Trombetti et al. 2016; Wu and Yeh 2016; Alex et al. 2013; Morris et al. 2010; Adler et al. 2009; Perrier et al. 2009; Repplinger et al. 2009; Esposito et al. 2008; Tsukahara et al. 2008; Caillard et al. 2007; Perrier et al. 2006; Roman et al. 2005; Quiros et al. 2003; Prager et al. 2002; Pasieka et al. 2002; Burney et al. 1998; Burney et al. 1996; McAllion and Paterson 1989; Numann et al. 1984). Joborn et al. (1988) were the first to set a focus on the importance of sleep disorders in patients with pHPT by the demonstration of a shortened sleep in such patients.

The pathophysiology of sleep disorders in pHPT is multifactorial. Possible reasons are in the first line all the symptoms connected with the disease, such as bone pain, myalgia, anxiety, and kidney stones. Another cause might be cardiac autonomic nerve dysfunction altering the circadian rhythm with an impact on sleep (Logue et al. 1990). Furthermore, the elevated PTH stimulates osteoblasts, which leads to an increase in interleukin-6 (IL-6) content that may reduce sleep efficiency. Elevated serum calcium reduces the regional cerebral blood flow by vasoconstriction, which may also cause sleep disorders. Autonomic dysfunction and biochemical changes characteristic of pHPT revert after parathyroidectomy when the PTH serum level normalizes (Murray et al. 2014; Mittendorf et al. 2007; Perrier et al. 2006; Safley et al. 2004; Mjäland et al. 2003; Nilsson et al. 2003).

Literature data on the impact of hyperparathyroidism on sleep quality and the effects of parathyroidectomy are scarce and contentious. Walker et al. (2004) and Joborn et al. (1989) have found insignificant changes in sleep quality after surgery. Contrarily, some other authors have found that sleep quality somehow improves after surgery (Friedman et al. 2005; Hong et al. 2005;

Opp 2005). Esposito et al. (2008) have reported an extension of patients' sleep time after surgery. These authors also report a high prevalence of sleep disorders in pHPT before surgery, reaching 95.5% of patients. We have previously demonstrated significant amelioration of cognitive functions in pHPT patients after parathyroidectomy (Dotzenrath et al. 2006), the finding recently confirmed by Shah-Becker et al. (2017). The present study expands on those findings by investigating the prevalence of sleep disorders in pHPT and the effects of parathyroidectomy on sleep quality. Using the PSQI questionnaire, we found a 70% prevalence of sleep disorders in pHPT patients before surgery. This figure is higher than the 25–30% estimated in the general population (DGSM 2015; DGSM 2009). Six months after parathyroidectomy, the prevalence was reduced to 54%. Statistically, the reduction was not significant, with the prevalence of sleep disorders remaining elevated when compared to the general population. However, we found that two specific sleep quality components, sleep latency and efficiency, significantly improved after parathyroidectomy. The score of the former decreased and the latter increased. The improvements are in line with a better quality of sleep after surgery.

In the present study, we did not notice changes in the other PSQI items such as sleep duration, sleep-disturbing events, the use of sleep medication, and daytime sleepiness and fatigue. The lack of changes in sleep duration is in line with the findings of Walker et al. (2004) and Joborn et al. (1989) but contrasts the elongation of sleep duration observed by Esposito et al. (2008). There is, however, a notion that sleep duration may not be a good reflection of impaired sleep quality (DGSM 2009). Sleep latency and efficiency are the essential features of sleep. Neither do patients with pHPT commonly suffer from excessive daytime sleepiness, characteristic of sleep-disordered breathing (Pasieka et al. 2009).

The clinical consequence is that patients with pHPT should be systematically questioned about the presence of sleep disorders, especially insomnia rather than hypersomnia. The presence of insomnia-impaired sleep might be an additional indication for performing parathyroidectomy. Vice versa, it should be considered to test patients without pHPT but suffering from insomnia for the presence of pHPT.

Acknowledgments The presented data are part of the doctoral thesis of Renan Viola Rasche of the Medical Faculty of the Heinrich-Heine-Universität, Düsseldorf, Germany, 2019.

Conflicts of Interest The authors declare no conflicts of interest concerning this chapter.

Ethical Approval All procedures performed in studies involving human participants were in accord with the ethical standards of the institutional and/or national research committee and with the 1964 Helsinki declaration and its later amendments or comparable ethical standards. The study was approved by the Ethics Committee of the Medical Faculty of the University of Witten/Herdecke, Germany.

Informed Consent Written informed consent was obtained from all individual participants included in the study.

References

Adler JT, Sippel RS, Schaefer S, Chen H (2009) Surgery improves quality of life in patients with "mild" hyperparathyroidism. Am J Surg 197(3):284–290

Alex G, Morris L, Pasieka J, Perrier N (2013) Nonclassical symptoms of primary hyperparathyroidism and their response to parathyroidectomy. Am Surg 79 (4):337–343

Burney RE, Jones KR, Coon JW, Blewitt DK, Herm AM (1996) Assessment of patient outcomes after operation for primary hyperparathyroidism. Surgery 120 (6):1013–1018

Burney RE, Jones KR, Peterson M, Christy B, Thompson NW (1998) Surgical correction of primary hyperparathyroidism improves quality of life. Surgery 124 (6):987–991

Buysee DJ, Reynolds CF 3rd, Monk TH, Bermann SR, Kupfer DJ (1989) The Pittsburgh Sleep Quality Index: a new instrument for psychiatric practice and research. Psychiatry Res 28(2):193–213

Caillard C, Sebag F, Mathonnet M, Gibelin H, Brunaud L, Loudot C, Kraimps JL, Hamy A, Bresler L, Charbonnel B, Leborgne J, Henry JF, Nguyen JM, Mirallié E (2007) Prospective evaluation of quality of life (SF-36v2) and nonspecific symptoms before and after cure of primary hyperparathyroidism (1-year follow-up). Surgery 141(2):153–159

DGSM (2007a) Deutsche Gesellschaft für Schlafforschung und Schlafmedizin. Fachinformationen. Fragebögen PSQI, Anleitung zur Handauswertung. Update 19 July 2007. https://www.dgsm.de/fachinformationen_frageboegen_psqi.php. Accessed 15 Jan 2021

DGSM (2007b) Deutsche Gesellschaft für Schlafforschung und Schlafmedizin. Fachinformationen. Fragebögen Epworth-Schläfrigkeitsskala. Update 19 July 2007. https://www.dgsm.de/fachinformationen_frageboegen_epworth.php?language=german. Accessed on 15 Jan 2021

DGSM (2009) S3-Leitlinie. Nicht erholsamer Schlaf/Schlafstörungen. Somnologie 13(Suppl 1):4–160. https://doi.org/10.1007/s11818-009-0430-8; https://www.dgzs.de/_downloads/s3-leitlinie-schlafstoerungen.pdf. Accessed on 15 Jan 2021

DGSM (2015) Deutsche Gesellschaft für Schlafforschung und Schlafmedizin. Fachinformationen. RKI-Bericht-Schlafstörungen. Update 2 February 2015. https://www.dgsm.de/fachinformationen_rki-bericht.php?language=germa. Accessed on 15 Jan 2021

Dotzenrath CM, Kaetsch AK, Pfingsten H, Cupisti K, Weyerbrock N, Vossough A, Verde PE, Ohmann C (2006) Neuropsychiatric and cognitive changes after surgery for primary hyperparathyroidism. World J Surg 30(5):680–685

Esposito MG, Cesare C, De Santo RM, Cice G, Perna AF, Violetti E, Conzo G, Bilancio G, Celsi S, Annunziata F, Iannelli S, De Santo NG, Cirillo M, Livrea A (2008) Parathyroidectomy improves the quality of sleep in maintenance hemodialysis patients with severe hyperparathyroidism. J Nephrol 21(Suppl 13): S92–S96

Friedman EM, Hayney MS, Love GD, Urry HL, Rosenkranz MA, Davidson SBH, Ryff CD (2005) Social relationships, sleep quality, and interleukin-6 in aging women. Proc Natl Acad Sci U S A 102 (51):18758–18762

Hong S, Mills PJ, Loredo JS, Adler KA, Dimsdale JE (2005) The association between interleukin-6, sleep, and demographic characteristics. Brain Behav Immun 19(2):165–172

Joborn C, Hetta J, Johansson H, Rastad J, Agren H, Akerström G, Ljunghall S (1988) Psychiatric morbidity in primary hyperparathyroidism. World J Surg 12 (4):476–481

Joborn C, Hetta J, Lind L, Rastad J, Akerström G, Ljunghall S (1989) Self-rated psychiatric symptoms in patients operated on because of primary hyperparathyroidism and in patients with longstanding mild hypercalcemia. Surgery 105(1):72–78

Kearns AE, Espiritu RP, Vickers Douglass K, Thapa P, Wermers RA (2019) Clinical characteristics and depression score response after parathyroidectomy in primary hyperparathyroidism. Clin Endocrinol 3:464–470

Liu JY, Peine BS, Mlaver E, Patel SG, Weber CJ, Saunders ND, Pofahl WE, Sharma J (2020) Neuropsychologic changes in primary hyperparathyroidism after parathyroidectomy from a dual-institution prospective study. Surgery 169(1):114–119

Logue FC, Fraser WD, Gallacher SJ, Cameron DA, O'Reilly DS, Beastall GH, Patel U, Boyle IT (1990) The loss of circadian rhythm for intact parathyroid hormone and nephrogenous cyclic AMP in patients with primary hyperparathyroidism. Clin Endocrinol 32(4):475–483

Lundgren E, Ljunghall S, Akerström G, Hetta J, Mallmin H, Rastad H (1998) Case-control study on symptoms and signs of "asymptomatic" primary hyperparathyroidism. Surgery 124(6):980–985

McAllion SJ, Paterson CR (1989) Psychiatric morbidity in primary hyperparathyroidism. Postgrad Med J 65 (767):628–631

Miedlich S, Koch CA, Paschke R (2002) Primärer Hyperparathyreoidismus: Heute ein meist asymptomatisches Krankheitsbild. Dtsch Arztebl 99: A3340–A3346

Mittendorf EA, Wefel JS, Meyers CA, Doherty D, Shapiro SE, Lee JE, Evans DB, Perrier ND (2007) Improvement of sleep disturbance and neurocognitive function after parathyroidectomy in patients with primary hyperparathyroidism. Endocr Pract 13:338–344

Mjäland O, Normann E, Halvorsen E, Rynning S, Egeland T (2003) Regional cerebral blood flow in patients with primary hyperparathyroidism before and after successful parathyroidectomy. Br J Surg 90(6):732–737

Morris GS, Grubbs EG, Hearon CM, Gantea S, Lee JE, Evans DB (2010) Parathyroidectomy improves functional capacity in "asymptomatic" older patients with primary hyperparathyroidism: a randomized control trial. Ann Surg 251(5):832–837

Murray SE, Pathak PR, Schaefer SC, Chen H, Sippel RS (2014) Improvement of sleep disturbance and insomnia following parathyroidectomy for primary hyperparathyroidism. World J Surg 38(3):542–548

Nilsson IL, Aberg J, Rastad J, Lind J (2003) Circadian cardiac autonomic nerve dysfunction in primary hyperparathyroidism improves after parathyroidectomy. Surgery 134(6):1013–1019

Numann PJ, Torppa AJ, Blumetti AE (1984) Neuropsychologic deficits with primary hyperparathyroidism. Surgery 96(6):1119–1123

Opp MR (2005) Cytokines and sleep. Sleep Med Rev 9 (5):355–364

Pasieka JL, Parsons LL, Demeure MJ, Wilson S, Malycha P, Jones J, Krzywda B (2002) Patient-based surgical outcome tool demonstrating alleviation of symptoms following parathyroidectomy in patients with primary hyperparathyroidism. World J Surg 26 (8):942–949

Pasieka JL, Parsons L, Jones J (2009) The long-term benefit of parathyroidectomy in primary hyperparathyroidism: a 10-year prospective surgical outcome study. Surgery 146(6):1006–10013

Perrier ND, Coker LH, Rorie KD, Burbank NS, Kirkland KA, Passmore LV, Tembreull T, Stump DA, Laurienti

PJ (2006) Preliminary report: functional MRI of the brain may be the ideal tool for evaluating neuropsychologic and sleep complaints of patients with primary hyperparathyroidism. World J Surg 30:686–696

Perrier ND, Balachandran D, Wefel JS, Jimenez C, Busaidy N, Morris GS, Dong W, Jackson E, Weaver S, Gantela S, Evans DB, Grubbs EG, Lee JE (2009) Prospective, randomized, controlled trial of parathyroidectomy versus observation in patients with "asymptomatic" primary hyperparathyroidism. Surgery 146(6):1116–1122

Prager G, Kalaschek A, Kaczirek K, Passler C, Scheuba C, Sonneck G, Niederle B (2002) Parathyroidectomy improves concentration and retentiveness in patients with primary hyperparathyroidism. Surgery 132 (6):930–935

Quiros RM, Alef MJ, Wilhelm SM, Djuicin G, Loviscek K, Prinz RA (2003) Health-related quality of life in hyperparathyroidism measurably improves after parathyroidectomy. Surgery 134(4):675–681

Repplinger D, Schaefer S, Chen H, Sippler RS (2009) Neurocognitive dysfunction: a predictor of parathyroid hyperplasia. Surgery 146(6):1138–1143

Roman SA, Sosa JA, Mayes L, Desmond E, Boudourakis L, Lin R, Snyder PJ, Holt E, Udelsman R (2005) Parathyroidectomy improves neurocognitive deficits in patients with primary hyperparathyroidism. Surgery 138(6):1121–1128

Safley SA, Villinger F, Jackson EH, Tucker-Burden C, Cohen C, Weber CJ (2004) Interleukin-6 production and secretion by human parathyroids. Clin Exp Immunol 136(1):145–156

Shah-Becker S, Derr J, Oberman BS, Baker A, Saunders B, Carr MM, Goldenberg D (2017) Early neurocognitive improvements following parathyroidectomy for primary hyperparathyroidism. Laryngoscope 128(3):775–780

Trombetti A, Christ ER, Henzen C, Gold G, Brändle M, Herrmann FR, Torriani C, Triponez F, Kraenzlin M, Rizzoli R, Meier C (2016) Clinical presentation and management of patients with primary hyperparathyroidism of the Swiss Primary Hyperparathyroidism Cohort: a focus on neuro-behavioral and cognitive symptoms. J Endocrinol Investig 39(5):567–576

Tsukahara K, Sugitani I, Fujimoto Y, Kawabata K (2008) Surgery did not improve the subjective neuropsychological symptoms of patients with incidentally detected mild primary hyperparathyroidism. Eur Arch Otorhinolaryngol 265(5):565–569

Walker RP, Paloyan E, Gopalsami C (2004) Symptoms in patients with primary hyperparathyroidism: muscle weakness or sleepiness. Endocr Pract 10(5):404–408

Weber T, Keller M, Hense I, Pietsch A, Hinz U, Schilling T, Nawroth P, Klar E, Büchler MW (2007) Effect of parathyroidectomy on quality of life and neuropsychological symptoms in primary hyperparathyroidism. World J Surg 31(6):1202–1209

Wu JX, Yeh MW (2016) Asymptomatic primary hyperparathyroidism: diagnostic pitfalls and surgical intervention. Surg Oncol Clin N Am 25(1):77–90

Adv Exp Med Biol - Clinical and Experimental Biomedicine (2022) 13: 129–135
https://doi.org/10.1007/5584_2021_632

Published online: 14 March 2021

Mini Craniotomy in the Management of Supratentorial Spontaneous Intracranial Hemorrhage: A Single-Center Outcome of the Minimally Invasive Treatment

Binod Bhattarai, Aliza Bajracharya, Suja Gurung, Sweta Giri, Sashi Bhusan Sah, and Sunil Munakomi

Abstract

Hemorrhagic stroke accounts for a significant proportion of mortality and confers a poor quality of life with high dependency among survivors. Surgical evacuation of hematoma has the advantage of rapidly controlling the increased intracranial pressure, halting the ongoing herniation syndrome, and mitigating the secondary cascades of events mediated by the inflammatory and blood degradation products. The advantage is hindered by the concurrent insult to the healthy brain tissue while passing through the normal brain tissue. Therefore, minimally invasive approaches to evacuate the hematoma are employed, but the need for an expensive surgical armamentarium and the expert multidisciplinary team is the bottleneck for their application, particularly in low-income nations. We herein performed a study upon the role of mini craniotomy open surgical method of evacuating hematoma in selected patients with supratentorial intracerebral hemorrhage. We found a significant reduction in the surgery length, minimized risk of post-surgery complications, shortened intensive care unit stay, and reduced mortality compared to the full-fledged craniotomy and endoscopy-guided surgery. There is a need for a large-scale randomized multicenter prospective study to verify the advantages of minimally invasive approaches in the management of symptomatic supratentorial intracerebral hemorrhages.

Keywords

Brain · Craniotomy · Hematoma · Intracerebral hemorrhage · Minimally invasive surgery · Mortality

B. Bhattarai, S. B. Sah, and S. Munakomi (✉)
Department of Neurosurgery, College of Medical Sciences, Bharatpur, Chitwan, Nepal
e-mail: neurobinod@gmail.com; sbhushanshah@gmail.com; sunilmunakomi@gmail.com

A. Bajracharya and S. Gurung
Department of Neurosurgery, Nobel Teaching Hospital, Morang, Nepal
e-mail: bajracharyaaliza@gmail.com; gurungsujakgbs@gmail.com

S. Giri
Department of Anesthesia, College of Medical Sciences, Bharatpur, Chitwan, Nepal
e-mail: Sg401564@gmail.com

1 Introduction

Spontaneous intracerebral hemorrhage is responsible for 9–27% of all strokes (Feigin et al. 2009). The mortality rate within 30 days has been reported to be as high as about 30% (Smajlović et al. 2008). Long-term survivors are often saddled with permanent deficits, with up to 75% suffering a significant disability. Surgical intervention is recommended for patients with a clot volume from 20 mL to 80 mL, worsening neurological status in relatively young patients, and hemorrhage causing midline brain shift or raised intracranial pressure (Siddique and Mendelow 2000). Various surgical strategies have been described ranging from craniotomies, decompressive surgery, to minimally invasive modalities like a stereotactic or endoscopic-aided aspiration. Craniotomy or decompressive large craniectomy facilitates good evacuation of hematoma and ensures effective hemostasis. However, the morbidity associated with general anesthesia, prolonged surgery duration, and blood loss is the inherent limitations. In minimally invasive procedures, the morbidity of extensive craniotomy can be obviated. Conventional craniotomy has a high mortality rate of 22–36%. Minimally invasive procedures have a high evacuation rate, low incidence of complication, better protection of normal neural tissue, and fewer surgery-related injuries. Direct visualization of bleeding points and coagulation of the responsible vessels also is feasible. The incidence of infectious complications is low, skin incisions are smaller, and surgery and intensive care unit stay are shorter (Zhang et al. 2014). Minimal invasiveness also encompasses collateral economic benefits, which plays an essential role in the health sector of low-to-middle income nations. The endoscopy-assisted evacuation of intracerebral hematoma is associated with a minimal rebleeding, reaching a meager 0–3.3% when compared to the 5–10% of the classical craniotomy approach (Gaab 2011). Minimally invasive procedures, however, require sophisticated and expensive armamentariums and the expert staff team for conducting specialized procedures such as endoscopy with neuro-navigation and catheter drainage. This study presents clinical outcomes in patients with spontaneous intracerebral hemorrhage treated with mini craniotomy in a tertiary hospital in Nepal. Minimally invasive surgery was performed with rather limited resources based on standard neurosurgical instruments, optimized direct visualization, and was aided with controlled brain retraction.

2 Methods

2.1 Patients

Eighty-five stroke patients, aged 52 ± 9 (M/F – 69/16), with lobar cortical and basal ganglia hemorrhages, treated with the minimally invasive approach of mini craniotomy in a tertiary hospital in Nepal were included in the study. A volume of hematoma was calculated from computer tomography (CT) images according to Kothari et al.'s (1996) formula. The specific anatomical site of the basal ganglionic hemorrhage was set according to Chung et al.'s (2000) localization scheme.

Inclusion criteria were as follows:

- Patient's age above 15
- CT scan showing spontaneous lobar or basal ganglia hemorrhage.
- Hematoma volume ≥ 30 mL
- Glasgow Coma Scale (GCS) motor score on admission ≥4 points

Exclusion criteria were as follows:

- Hemorrhage caused by secondary factors like vascular malformations, tumors, or head injury
- Features of advanced herniation with infarction seen in the neuroradiologic examination
- GCS motor score on admission <4 points
- Multiple intracranial hemorrhages
- Clotting disorders
- Preexisting neurological deficits like previous intracerebral hematoma or infarct
- Gross ventricular enlargement
- Consent refusal

2.2 Sample Size Calculation

The minimum statistically meaningful sample size of patients for this study was calculated using the formula:

$$N = z^2 \, x \, p \, x \, q / d^2$$

where $Z = 1.96$ at 95% confidence interval

p = prevalence of hemorrhagic stroke taken as 30%
q = 1-p
d = margin of error taken as 10%

The result of the calculation was 80.8, and we included 85 patients in the study.

Overall, we recorded and evaluated the following elements: clinical and radiological outcomes, demographic data, hematoma volume, GCS on admission, duration of the surgical procedure, intraoperative and postoperative complications, and duration of stay in the intensive care unit (ICU) after surgery.

2.3 Surgical Approach

Surgery was performed under endotracheal general anesthesia. A linear skin incision was made. Mini craniotomy of 2.0–2.5 cm in diameter over a frontal or skull parietal area was depending on the shortest way to the epicenter of a hematoma. A cruciate dural opening followed by a small corticotomy was made over the relatively non-eloquent area. The hematoma was then evacuated using controlled suction aided with biopsy forceps to mince the hematoma. Hemostasis was achieved by continuous saline irrigation, pressure packing, using a bipolar cautery, and standard micro-neurosurgical techniques. The hematoma cavity was lined with fibrin sealant and the dura was left open and covered with gel foam. The bone was repositioned. The scalp was then closed in layers.

3 Results

Clinical features of hemorrhagic stroke patients are shown in Table 1. Although a documented history of arterial hypertension was present in 71 (83.5%) patients, compliance with antihypertensive treatment, the therapy was seen in only about one-third of them. The proportion of basal ganglia and cortical lobar bleeds was 3 to 1. In basal ganglia, the anatomically lateral variant was the most common hemorrhage site in 38 (59.4%) out of the 64 patients, followed by the massive hemorrhage in 19 out of the 64 (29.7%) patients, and the anterior variant in 7 (10.9%) out of the 64 patients. The mean volume of hematoma was 46.5 ± 10.5(SD) mL, the mean duration of the surgical procedure was 36.5 min, and the mean post-surgery time spent in the ICU was 3.2 ± 0.8 days. A difficulty in achieving hemostasis deep inside the hematoma cavity was seen in 2 cases only and the rebleeding occurred in 3 (3.8%) out of the 85 patients with re-evacuation carried out in 2 of them. Three (3.8) patients died, with pulmonary embolism accounting for two deaths and ventriculitis for one.

The mini craniotomy bone flap and the post-operative CT-reconstructed 3D skull image are schematically illustrated in Fig. 1. Representative examples of preoperative and postoperative CT images of the cortical and basal ganglia hemorrhage sites are demonstrated in Fig. 2.

4 Discussion

Primary injury caused by spontaneous intracerebral hemorrhage is mainly due to the mechanical mass effect of a hematoma. Secondary injuries are triggered by the developing inflammation and degraded blood products. The prime benefit of surgical evacuation is the rapid control of increased intracranial pressure, which mitigates the harmful cascade of cerebral herniation,

Table 1 Clinical features

Age (years)	52 ± 9
Male/female ratio	69/16; 4.3:1.0
History of hypertension (n)	71 (83.5%)
Compliance with antihypertensive medications (n)	30 (35.3%)
Mean volume of hematoma (mL)	46.5 ± 10.5
Basal ganglia/cortical bleeds ratio	64/21; 3:1
Anatomic distribution of basal ganglia bleeds	Anterior –7/64 (10.9%) Lateral – 38/64 (59.4%) Massive – 19/64 (29.7%)
Duration of surgical procedure (min)	36.5 ± 5.2
Complications	Rebleeding -3/85 (3.8%) Mortality - 3/85 (3.8%)
Duration of stay in the intensive care unit (days)	3.2 ± 0.8

Mean data are ±SD

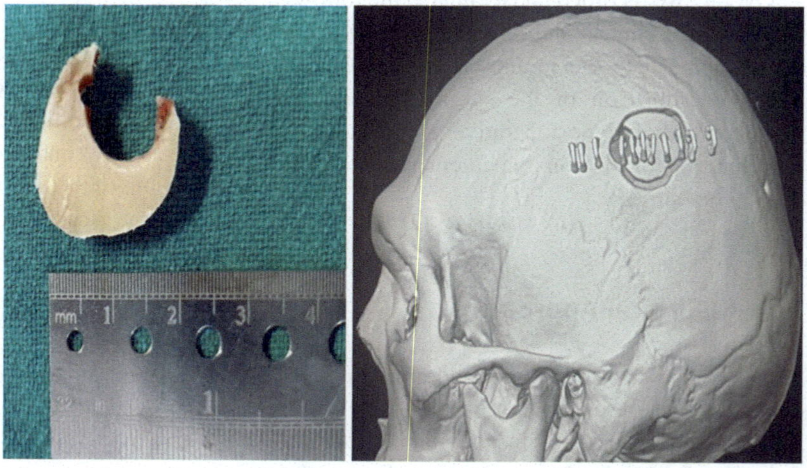

Fig. 1 A mini craniotomy bone flap and the post-operative computer tomography reconstructed skull image

restores cerebral perfusion, and inhibits the development of inflammation (Gaab 2011). The recent progress in minimally invasive surgical techniques to treat intracerebral hematoma, like endoscopy-guided stereotactic aspiration, is advantageous in that the inescapable trauma to the normal brain tissue is minimized and the clot hematoma is rapidly evacuated. A small surgical wound and limited intraoperative blood loss make wound healing better. Further, shortened surgery duration in relatively stable patients promotes early extubation, decreases the odds of postoperative pulmonary complications, and reduces the duration of patient stay in the ICU, all of which is conducive to faster patient recuperation and post-surgery rehabilitation.

Nonetheless, the control of bleeding and proper manipulation of instruments in the restrained operational space are limiting factors in minimally invasive surgical procedures that require much training and expertise (Ratre et al. 2018). The cost factor associated with the use of such methods also plays a role in low-to-middle income nations. The financial burden accounts for a significant proportion of "leave against medical advice", i.e., abandoning useful medical procedures (Hasan et al. 2019). An incomplete clot evacuation is another major concern. Classical craniotomy has an obvious advantage of decreasing the raised intracranial pressure along with the evacuation of a hematoma. The minimal approaches lag on this account, and there is a risk

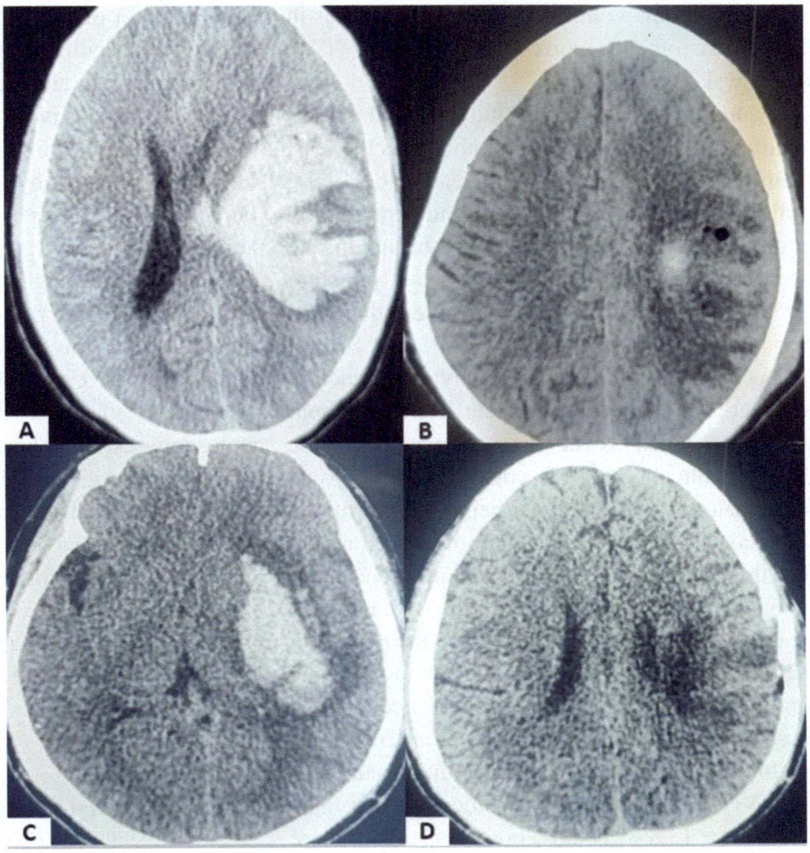

Fig. 2 Representative examples of preoperative and postoperative computer tomography images of cortical (panel A and B) and basal ganglia (panel C and D) hemorrhage sites

of brain edema in a subset of patients despite hematoma evacuation, necessitating the need for conversion to a larger craniotomy. A minimally invasive technique would not be recommended in patients with a low Glasgow Coma Scale score, moribund neurological status, and clinico-radiological features of advanced brain herniation. The minimal approach sometimes has a limitation of ensuring hemostasis, especially at the depth of a cavity, or complete hematoma removal concurrent with the minimum brain retraction. The technical difficulty of appropriate surgical light focusing at the depth of a cavity also is a major concern. In the present study, we thoroughly assessed the practical feasibility of performing the minimally invasive procedure for intracranial hematoma evacuation in a selected group of stroke patients. We herein report that the procedure can be safely undertaken with the application of basic neurosurgical instruments, fulfilling the required criteria of surgical treatment of the ailment, with add-on advantages of less surgical insult to the brain, less anesthesia, and perioperative patient stress, and faster recuperation.

A higher proportion of male patients were found to suffer from spontaneous intracranial hemorrhage in the present study, which is in line with some of the previous reports (Khallaf and Abdelrahman 2019). However, the gender predominance of brain hematoma is a contentious issue as some other reports point to a similar incidence rate in both sexes (van Asch et al. 2010; Appelros et al. 2009). The most common location of a spontaneous brain bleed among both conservatively and surgically managed patients is the basal ganglia area (Rychen et al. 2020). We confirmed the predominance of basal ganglia in the present study with 75.3% of patients having a hemorrhagic stroke in this area. Likewise, the mean hematoma volume of 46 mL we found is in line with other reports (Luan et al. 2019; Rutkowski et al. 2019).

A previous comparative study showed a minimally invasive puncture and drainage as the least traumatic procedure with the least blood loss, followed by the endoscopy and craniotomy groups. However, the hematoma evacuation rate was lower in the minimally invasive puncture group (35.2%) compared with the other two groups where it amounted to 90.8% and 87.3%, respectively. Yet the minimally invasive puncture enjoyed the shortest treatment time of about 38 min, which is far less compared to the 98–120 min of the endoscopy-assisted removal of hematoma, with the latter being one-fourth the time taken for the classical craniotomy approach. On the downside, the minimally invasive puncture had the highest rebleeding rate. By contrast, a craniotomy was more effective in removing hematoma but resulted in marked trauma to the brain and also has the highest incidence of post-surgery pulmonary infection (Fu et al. 2019).

In the present study, the rebleeding occurred in just 3 (3.8%) out of the 85 patients. There also were three (3.8%) deaths. For comparison, there were 6 deaths out of the 40 (15%) patients and 4 out of the 25 (16%) patients undergoing minimally invasive craniotomy reported in the studies of Luan et al. (2019) and Rutkowski et al. (2019), respectively. Concerning other studies and other treatment modalities, data on the mortality rate are divergent. A study by Fu et al. (2019) has reported a mortality rate of 1.6% in the endoscopy-assisted management of intracranial hemorrhage, 3.6% in the minimally invasive puncture, and 5.0% in the craniotomy groups. By contrast, much higher mortality rates have been reported by Ratre et al. (2018) amounting to 11% in patients undergoing the endoscopy-assisted management of spontaneous bleed into the basal ganglia area and by Rychen et al. (2020) amounting to 21.3% in craniotomy with hematoma evacuation.

Pulmonary post-surgery embolism is a rare but mortal event. In this study, we noticed two such fatalities compared to one case in a study by Luan et al. (2019). We also noticed two (2.3%) cases of inflammation of the ependymal lining, with one of the ventriculitis being fatal. Surgical site infections are another leading cause of mortality among stroke survivors (Kuohn et al. 2020).

In conclusion, mini craniotomy evacuation of hematoma caused by spontaneous intracranial hemorrhage in patients suitable for this kind of surgery showed good clinical outcomes, minimizing the length of a surgical procedure, intraoperative and postoperative complications, length of stay in the ICU, and mortality rate when compared to reports on other treatment modalities such as classical craniotomy or endoscopy-assisted hematoma evacuation. The minimized surgical site infection and a shorter stay in the intensive care unit as seen in our patients promotes the "patient care bundle" approach by facilitating early rehabilitative programs. The relative ease of performing the procedure with basic neurosurgical instruments calls for the appraisal and validation of these findings in randomized multicenter prospective studies.

Conflicts of Interest The authors declare no conflicts of interest concerning this article.

Ethical Approval All procedures performed in studies involving human participants were in accord with the ethical standards of the institutional and/or national research committee and with the 1964 Helsinki declaration and its later amendments or comparable ethical standards. The study was approved by the Institutional Review Committee of the College of Medical Sciences in Chitwan, Nepal; permit no. 2020-107.

Informed Consent Written informed consent was obtained from all individual participants included in the study or their guardians.

References

Appelros P, Stegmayr B, Terent A (2009) Sex differences in stroke epidemiology: a systematic review. Stroke 40 (4):1082–1090

Chung CS, Caplan LR, Yamamoto Y, Chang HM, Lee SJ, Song HJ, Lee HS, Shin HK, Yoo KM (2000) Striatocapsular haemorrhage. Brain 123 (Pt 9):1850–1862

Feigin VL, Lawes CM, Bennett DA, Barker-Collo SL, Parag V (2009) Worldwide stroke incidence and early case fatality reported in 56 population-based studies: a systematic review. Lancet Neurol 8(4):355–369

Fu CH, Wang N, Chen B, Wang P, Chen H, Liu W, Liu L (2019) Surgical management of moderate basal ganglia intracerebral hemorrhage: comparison of safety and efficacy of endoscopic surgery, minimally invasive puncture and drainage, and craniotomy. World Neurosurg 122:e995–e1001

Gaab MR (2011) Intracerebral hemorrhage (ICH) and intraventricular hemorrhage (IVH): improvement of bad prognosis by minimally invasive neurosurgery. World Neurosurg 75(2):206–208

Hasan O, Samad MA, Khan H, Sarfraz M, Noordin S, Ahmad T, Nowshad G (2019) Leaving against medical advice from in-patients departments rate, reasons and predicting risk factors for re-visiting hospital retrospective cohort from a tertiary care hospital. Int J Health Policy Manag 8(8):474–479

Khallaf M, Abdelrahman M (2019) Surgical management for large hypertensive basal ganglionic hemorrhage: single center experience. Egypt J Neurosurg 34(1):19

Kothari RU, Brott T, Broderick JP, Barsan WG, Sauerbeck LR, Zuccarello M, Khoury J (1996) The ABCs of measuring intracerebral hemorrhage volumes. Stroke 27(8):1304–1305

Kuohn LR, Leasure AC, Acosta JN, Vanent K, Murthy SB, Kamel H, Matouk CC, Sansing LH, Falcone GJ, Sheth KN (2020) Cause of death in spontaneous intracerebral hemorrhage survivors: multistate longitudinal study. Neurology 95(20):e2736–e2745

Luan L, Li M, Sui H, Li G, Pan W (2019) Efficacies of minimally invasive puncture and small bone window craniotomy for hypertensive intracerebral hemorrhage, evaluation of motor-evoked potentials and comparison of postoperative rehemorrhage between the two methods. Exp Ther Med 17(2):1256–1261

Ratre S, Yadav N, Parihar VS, Dubey A, Yadav YR (2018) Endoscopic surgery of spontaneous basal ganglionic hemorrhage. Neurol India 66(6):1694–1703

Rutkowski M, Song I, Mack W, Zada G (2019) Outcomes after minimally invasive parafascicular surgery for intracerebral hemorrhage: a single-center experience. World Neurosurg 132:e520–e528

Rychen J, O'Neill A, Lai LT, Bervini D (2020) Natural history and surgical management of spontaneous intracerebral hemorrhage: a systematic review. J Neurosurg Sci 64(6):558–570

Siddique SM, Mendelow AD (2000) Surgical treatment of intracerebral haemorrhage. Br Med Bull 56 (2):444–456

Smajlović D, Salihović D, Ibrahimagić OC, Sinanović O, Vidović M (2008) Analysis of risk factors, localization and 30-day prognosis of intracerebral hemorrhage. Bosn J Basic Med Sci 8(2):121–125

van Asch CJ, Luitse MJ, Rinkel GJ, van der Tweel I, Algra A, Klijn CJ (2010) Incidence, case fatality, and functional outcome of intracerebral haemorrhage over time, according to age, sex, and ethnic origin: a systematic review and meta-analysis. Lancet Neurol 9 (2):167–176

Zhang HZ, Li YP, Yan ZC, Wang XD, She L, Wang XD, Dong L (2014) Endoscopic evacuation of basal ganglia hemorrhage via keyhole approach using an adjustable cannula in comparison with craniotomy. Biomed Res Int 2014:898762–898762

Adv Exp Med Biol - Clinical and Experimental Biomedicine (2022) 13: C1
https://doi.org/10.1007/5584_2021_650

Published online: 10 June 2021

Correction to: Outcome of Repeat Pulmonary Metastasectomy

Marcus Krüger, Katharina Franzke, Taufiek Konrad Rajab, Fabian Nadler, Moritz Möbius-Winkler, Norman Zinne, Daniel Schulz, Miriam Möller, Wolfgang Schütte, Michael Ermitsch, Bassam Redwan, Olaf Schega, and Christian Biancosino

Correction to: Chapter "Outcome of Repeat Pulmonary Metastasectomy" in: Adv Exp Med Biol - Clinical and Experimental Biomedicine, https://doi.org/10.1007/5584_2021_635

The chapter was inadvertently published with an incorrect chapter title, which has now been corrected to read as "Outcome of Repeat Pulmonary Metastasectomy".

The updated version of this chapter can be found at https://doi.org/10.1007/5584_2021_635

The manufacturer's authorised representative in the EU is Springer Nature Customer Service Centre GmbH, Europaplatz 3, 69115 Heidelberg, Germany. If you have any concerns regarding our products, please contact ProductSafety@springernature.com

Printed and bound by CPI Group (UK) Ltd, Croydon, CR0 4YY
22/09/2026
02221063-0017